THE *very* GOOD NEWS
ABOUT WINE

Authoritative health evidence
the health authorities don't tell you

D1522822

Tony Edwards

In loving memory of my mother,
Hilda Edwards BSc, 1914-2004

Contents

The Author

Tony Edwards is a former BBC TV producer/ director/ writer, with over 80 science documentaries to his credit, some winning awards from such bodies as the British Medical Association. After the BBC, he wrote on science, technology and medicine for *The Sunday Times, Readers Digest, Daily Mail* and a wide variety of medical magazines. He is married to the broadcaster and novelist Debbie Rix; they have two grown-up children, three hens and four cats, and live in rural Kent.

Acknowledgements

My primary thanks are due to Sergey Brin and Larry Page for their financial support of Google Scholar, whose truly encyclopedic medical database has made this book possible.

I am also very pleased to thank Mr Said Abisi FRCS, Professor Ramon Estruch, Nicki Forrest, Dr Zoe Harcombe PhD, Dr Richard Harding PhD, Olivier Humbreck, Lalou Bize-Leroy, Hayo Loacker, Keith Ougden, and Professors Byron Sharp and Karol Sikora.

It goes without saying that I am entirely responsible for the book's contents.

Author's Note

This book attempts to distil the medical evidence from many hundreds of scientific studies about alcohol and health. In reporting the evidence, it occasionally draws inferences about their practical import for the individual. However, the book is essentially a reportage, and is not intended as health advice. Although the information and opinions provided here are believed to be accurate and sound, readers should make their own enquiries and/or consult knowledgeable health professionals before acting upon anything they read in this book.

The author and the publisher cannot be held responsible nor liable for any loss or claim arising from the use of the information in this book.

1

Introduction

This is my second book about alcohol and health. My first *The Good News About Booze** was published in late 2013, and I had no plans to write another. That book was, I felt, a sufficiently comprehensive assessment of the health effects of drinking – both positive and negative, despite its up-beat title. It summarised 50 years of medical evidence amply demonstrating two related but counter-intuitive discoveries: 1. drinking moderate amounts of alcohol is good for one's health, 2. drinking no alcohol at all can be almost as injurious to health as drinking too much.

So, exactly ten years later, why write another book on the same subject? What's the point of reiterating half a century's worth of data overwhelmingly pointing in the same direction? After all, since my first book, that evidence has not significantly changed. Most drinkers still live longer and healthier lives than teetotallers and serial drunkards.

What has changed, however, is the attitude to drinking taken by the 'medical authorities'. Year by year, the quantity of alcohol officially declared to be safe to drink has been reduced. In almost every country round the world, the 'alcohol guidelines' are now much lower than in 2013. For example, in 2016 the UK reduced its advised intake from 4 'units' of alcohol a day to 2, while marijuana-smoking Holland slashed theirs to 1 unit (a maiden aunt's glass of sherry) per day, and France shocked its *buveurs* by declaring that as little as a standard *quart de vin rouge* a day would send them to an early grave.

---

* Triggered by my chance discovery that alcohol does not put on weight.

1

That downbeat message has been reinforced by campaigns such as Dry January, initiated in 2014 by a cabal of British so-called 'alcohol charities'.

Understandably, many people now believe that alcohol is more harmful than was thought, and that it might be prudent to give it up altogether – as with tobacco. This has led to the development of low and zero alcohol beers and wines, and bizarrely even 100% alcohol-free spirits/liquor. This denaturing of liquids which humans have enjoyed for millennia has been paradoxically welcomed by both alcohol's friends and enemies. The medical authorities are pleased to see a decline in alcohol consumption, while the alcohol industry is delighted to be able to charge almost as much for its products as before, pocketing most of the tax previously levied on the alcohol contents.

And yet, to repeat, there is no new public health justification for these developments. The evidence continues to show that drinking alcohol within sensible limits has powerful health benefits. Alone, that's a good enough reason for writing this updated book, simply to counter the growing prohibitionist messages.

However, there's an even better reason – mainly about wine. Compared to a decade ago, there's stronger evidence not only that wine is exceptionally good for one's health, but also that its downsides had been exaggerated. It's now clear that wine drinking is not associated with some of the cancers it was once believed to be, and indeed that it may actually do the reverse. Yes, you read that right: quite a few cancers can be prevented by drinking wine.

That bombshell discovery is the meat of Chapter 2. Subsequent chapters cover the latest medical evidence for wine's benefits in the other major killers of our time – heart disease, diabetes, obesity and dementia.

Taken together, these findings are astonishing. Wine turns out to be far superior to most vitamin mineral/supplements, exercise regimes or pharmaceutical drugs. This explains why wine drinkers are among the longest-living and healthiest people on the planet.

Indeed, if wine were patentable, pharmaceutical companies would surely be producing tanker-loads of it to sell to health authorities, as a simple way to reduce the general burden of disease and the consequent pressure on health services. Something along these lines was already common as recently as 70 years ago. In the early days of Britain's National Health Service, general practitioners/ family physicians were allowed to prescribe wine medicinally, while hospitals routinely doled out sherry (fortified wine) to their in-patients. Equally, during the Prohibition era in 1920's USA, the easiest way to obtain wine legally was at a pharmacy, brandishing a doctor's prescription for your heart condition.*

Why the 21st century has seen such a dramatic medical volte-face is discussed in chapter 14, while by contrast, chapter 12 discusses the introduction of organic farming methods into viticulture, thus making wine even healthier by eliminating pesticide residues.

The book also opens up a fresh question: are the new alcohol-free wines as beneficial to health as the real liquid? Undoubtedly, one of the motivations to forego alcohol is based on the perceived health benefits of abstinence. But what's the actual evidence? Chapter 13 investigates this in some detail.

A warning about the book. Because its contents fly in the face of the 'authorised gospel' about alcohol and health, it behoves me to counter readers' understandable scepticism by providing 'chapter and verse' about the evidence. That entails delving fairly deeply into medical data. So it's not always an easy read, because the book cites literally hundreds of medical studies demonstrating that wine is beneficial to health, while also being up front about the relatively few that don't. If you

---

* The other way was to go to church. Christian ministers were allowed to dispense 'sacramental wine' during services. Unsurprisingly, Prohibition saw church attendances skyrocketing.

wish to skip the details, however, there is a summary at the end of every main chapter.

On the other hand, for readers prepared to wade through the science, I have tried to enliven the text with the odd bit of levity, occasional splashes of populist prose and use of the first person. But that should not detract from the book's serious dispassionate purpose: to inform people who already enjoy a few glasses of wine a day that their allegedly harmful pleasure is in fact quite the reverse, according to the published scientific evidence.

It is important for public health that any directives issued by the medical authorities should be challenged by the actual science. Alcohol, and wine in particular, exhibits this in spades. Nanny Stateism is already bad enough but a Nanny State which clearly - and probably knowingly - deceives its people is intolerable.

A note about the amounts of alcohol quoted in the book. Because alcohol 'units' are confusing and rarely used in modern medical journals, I have employed the accepted scientific measure of alcohol quantities: grams. As a rough guide, **a bottle of wine contains about 80 grams of alcohol, a pint of beer 20, and a measure of spirits/liquor 12 grams.** It would help you to make a mental note of these figures - although I often include reminders in the text.

Nothing in the book should be taken as medical advice, however. Readers who wish to act upon its contents should satisfy themselves of their veracity, or take advice from knowledgeable health professionals (sadly a very rare breed).

A final word about the title. Although the book focusses on wine, it inevitably covers the health effects of alcohol in general, so it will also be of interest to drinkers of beer, brandy, gin, rum, saké, sherry, whisky, vodka, and all the other alcoholic drinks which enliven many people's lives.

2

The Big C

Cancer, the most feared of diseases, and therefore the one that the medical authorities like to scare us with when dishing the dirt on drink – as they so often do.

In fact, no less a body than the International Agency for Research on Cancer (part of the World Health Organisation) now classifies alcohol as a "Class 1 carcinogen", thus putting it in the same category as tobacco and asbestos. In other words, officialdom says drinking will significantly increase your risk of cancer – no question.

But in fact there are loads of questions about alcohol and cancer.

If you read the small print of many of the scientific papers on the subject, you'll find experts pointing out many "uncertainties" in the evidence – even to the extent of admitting that the data is often "contradictory."[1] But these major caveats about the alcohol/cancer evidence-base are never aired in public.

For example, there's another organisation called the World Cancer Research Fund (WCRF) which every few years publishes a report on all known causes of cancer. It is unequivocal in its condemnation of drinking - albeit somewhat tortuously expressed:

> There is no threshold for the level of (alcohol) consumption below which there is no increase in the risk of at least some cancers. For cancer prevention, it's best not to drink alcohol.[2]

Also, no bones about it, says the WCRF, wine is as hazardous as any other booze:

> Alcoholic drinks are a cause of various cancers, irrespective of the type of alcoholic drink consumed.[3]

But do such ex-cathedra statements from supposedly authoritative sources really stack up? Read on.

The Evidence

There's at least half a century of research data on the alcohol/cancer connection. Studied closely, they show that the actual evidence is often at variance with the grim cancer headlines generated by the authorities.

In a sentence, the rest of this chapter will show that drinking does indeed appear to be associated with some cancers, but that astonishingly it often *does the reverse* – particularly if you drink wine.

But don't get your hopes up too soon, as I'm kicking off with some bad news about wine and cancer.

Mouth, Throat and Gullet Cancers

Of all the cancers, these ('head and neck' cancers, in medspeak) are far and away the most obviously caused by alcohol. That's hardly surprising, as they're the parts of the body booze hits first, and where it's most vulnerable to alcohol's poisonous effects. By contrast, as we'll see in later chapters, once alcohol's got down into the stomach, the body starts a highly efficient detoxification process, using clever enzyme chemistry to turn poisonous alcohol into harmless acetic acid. But while alcohol is swilling past the lips and down through the mouth, throat and gullet, the body has little or no protection against it.

The people most at risk for getting cancer in these areas are the unfortunates (or fools, depending on your point of view) who both smoke and drink spirits/liquor. That combo can multiply cancer risk dramatically. [4] Why? Because tobacco smoke interacts with oral bacteria, turning alcohol into acetaldehyde, a suspected carcinogen.[5]

For example, the late Anglo-American writer Christopher Hitchens was a sad casualty to tobacco and liquor. However, if Hitch had quit smoking and chosen to drink a moderate amount of wine rather than spirits, he would probably still be alive today. And amazingly he might have actually reduced his risk of getting the cancer that killed him.

How come?

In the late 1990's a US study done under the auspices of the hugely prestigious National Cancer Institute made the astonishing discovery that wine drinkers have a *reduced risk* of the two main cancers of the gullet, compared to people who never touch a drop of alcohol – up to 20% less risk of squamous cell cancer, and a staggering 50% reduction for adenocarcinoma.[6]

However, the problem with studies done in the USA is that Americans are not huge wine-drinkers, so this dramatic reduction in gullet cancers only seems to apply at relatively low intakes.

For example, when you look at countries like Italy, where some people regularly drink a couple of bottles of wine a day, doctors have found a huge extra risk, calculating that at that intake, the extra risk of mouth and throat cancer is 11 times higher, and up to a staggering 18 times for esophageal cancer.[7] [8] These two risk figures are on a par with lung cancer and smoking, so serious wine bibbers need to take them seriously.

On the other hand, these high risks among Italians may be due to specific genetic differences within populations, says one study.[9] In fact, an Italian artist friend of mine sadly died of throat cancer in his mid-70s, despite being a non-smoker and only a modest wine drinker.

Nevertheless, a large international study does confirm that drinking a bottle of wine a day can raise your risk of these cancers by over six times - although again that extra risk is considerably enhanced among smokers.[10]

Paradoxically, however, at lower intakes, it's pretty clear that wine drinkers do have a reduced risk of the commonest cancer in this area of the body - the gullet. The clinching evidence has come from two separate research teams in the USA and Australia who have investigated a condition called Barrett's Esophagus (BE), an irritation of the lining of the gullet which is a major precursor of cancer. What did the research show? That if you drink a large glass of wine a day, you roughly halve your risk of BE compared to non-drinkers.[11] [12]

But what about wine drinkers who don't stick to such low intakes? Luckily, there's a simple but powerful solution: increase the intake of Vitamin B9, also known as folate. As it happens, one of the side-effects of alcohol is to reduce the body's store of folate – a valuable micronutrient found in leafy green vegetables, legumes, avocados and nuts. Lack of it is now known to be a risk factor for cancer in general, not just in drinkers.[13] The good news is that if their folate* levels are high enough, drinkers' extra risk of mouth, throat and gullet cancers drops dramatically, according to a plethora of international studies.[14] [15] [16] [17] [18]

So it makes sense for heavy wine drinkers to either beef up their intake of leafy green veggies etc., or pop a daily folate supplement.

Liver Cancer

If there's one organ that doctors always say alcohol is bad for, it's the liver, as it causes both liver cancer as well as cirrhosis.

Certainly, it's not unreasonable to presume the liver might be badly affected by alcohol: after all, booze is a toxin, and the liver is where all poisons – from pesticides to pharmaceuticals – get detoxified.

---

* Folate is not be confused with folic acid. Although they are chemically identical, the former is derived from plants, the latter is synthetic and less bioavailable.

So, few of us will be surprised by the idea that alcohol and livers don't mix. However, once again, it turns out that the scientific evidence is not as clear-cut as you might imagine.

First, researchers admit that many of the medical surveys are both "contradictory" and "not statistically significant", implying that if there is any liver cancer/drink connection at all, it must be pretty damn weak.[19]

And weak is the word. In 2014 Italian researchers tried to make sense of the jumble of disparate research findings, and finally came up with a cancer risk figure. They concluded that drinking up to the equivalent of half a bottle of wine a day has no liver cancer consequences at all. Double that intake does increase liver cancer risk, but only by a mere 22%.[20] I'll explain later why 22% isn't worth worrying about.

Liver Cirrhosis

When livers and alcohol mentioned, it's cirrhosis that people mostly think of – although, curiously enough, it wasn't until the 1970's that alcohol was discovered to cause it.[21]

Unlike the liver cancer evidence, however, the cirrhosis connection is cast-iron. There's consistent evidence that the more you drink, the greater your risk of cirrhosis – a so-called 'dose response', which is a causal clincher.[22]

Cirrhosis can be a precursor of cancer, as well as being potentially fatal in its own right, so it's the Number One health reason we're given for laying off the drink. Here's a quote from a 2013 report by European liver experts:

> Liver cirrhosis has... become a serious health threat in some Western European countries.... Alcohol has long been identified as the strongest risk factor for liver cirrhosis. In fact, cirrhosis mortality has traditionally been used as a valid indicator for tracing the health consequences of alcohol abuse.[23]

But just how serious is the cirrhosis problem, really? Here are the facts.

Much of the research on cirrhosis has come from Scandinavia where there's quite a lot of 'problem drinking', despite draconian alcohol taxes - and the upshot is that the cirrhosis threat is less than you might have thought.

In the 1980s, Danish researchers tracked the health of more than 13,000 people for over 12 years, specifically looking for a connection between drinking and Alcoholic Liver Disease (ALD: a catch-all term including both cirrhosis and liver cancer). As expected, they found that drinkers did have an extra risk of ALD.[24]

But crucially, this risk only applied to relatively few people. Fully 93% of drinkers had no signs of any liver problems whatever, even at alcohol intakes of around the equivalent of two bottles of wine a day.

Another Danish research group reported similar findings, after closely monitoring nearly three hundred heavy drinkers for 13 years to see how many developed ALD. The men were chosen specifically because they were all "alcohol abusing", and yet, once again, fewer than 7% of them developed cirrhosis.[25]

The next step up - or down, depending on your point of view – the alcohol ladder is full-blown alcoholism. Surely, most addicts must be riddled with cirrhosis, you would think. Well they're not, according to Swedish medics, who find that roughly 4 out of 5 of their alcoholics never succumb at all.[26]

That's not a freak Scandinavian finding, for in 2003 researchers at Canada's prestigious (and somewhat hawkish) Center for Addiction and Mental Health surveyed the entire international evidence and reported that:

> Alcoholics ...drink an average of 160 grams of undiluted alcohol per day. About 14 percent of alcoholics will develop cirrhosis if they drink this quantity for a period of 8 years.[27]

Let's look at these figures. 160 grams of neat alcohol is roughly the contents of a medium-sized bottle of spirits – a huge amount of hooch to down every single day. And yet here we have world experts telling us that 86% of drinkers can swallow that quantity, for years on end, and not get cirrhosis at all.

What about wine, though? After all, wine drinkers are rarely full-blown alcoholics – and vice versa.[28]

Yet again, the data reveal a bit of a paradox. Like other alcohols, wine can indeed cause cirrhosis, but unlike other alcohols it can also prevent it – a discovery first made in a huge long-term study by Danish scientists in 2004. However, it all depends on the dose: prevention occurs below moderate intakes - about a third of a bottle a day. Above that, the risk of cirrhosis rises, but much less steeply than with beer and spirits.[29]

But Denmark isn't the ideal place to assess wine and cirrhosis, simply because very few Danes are exclusive wine drinkers. Once again, a good place to find them is a thousand miles south in sunny Italy, one of the top wine-glugging countries in Europe, with a goodly number of heavy drinkers. In the 1990s a posse of concerned Italian liver experts descended on a couple of small towns in Northern Italy and began a detailed investigation of the inhabitants' drinking habits and liver problems – even to the extent of taking liver biopsies (ouch!) - fully expecting to find their countrymen riddled with disease. This wasn't the case, however. They found not a trace of cirrhosis in people who drank under a third of a bottle of wine a day – nor indeed any liver problems at all. But above that, they were surprised to discover that the risk didn't rise nearly as much as they expected:

> Even at the highest level of alcohol intake (over two bottles of wine a day), the percentage of people with alcohol-induced liver damage was relatively low at 13.5% [30]

In other words, almost 9 in 10 heavy drinkers had no liver problems whatsoever. An important aside: people who drank wine only at mealtimes had even less risk of liver damage.

Puzzled by the very low rates of liver disease in heavy drinkers, another posse of Italian experts descended on the same two towns, armed with genetic-testing kits. They found that cirrhosis tended to occur in people with unusual variants of the two enzymes responsible for detoxifying alcohol in the liver, pointing out that these genetic variants are "very low in Caucasians".[31]

In fact, the evidence suggests that if you're unlucky enough to have the wrong genes, you may get liver disease almost no matter how little you drink.[32] Fortunately, most of us seem to have the right genes, which may explain why most drinkers don't get liver disease.

Bowel Cancer

This cancer of the colon and rectum (hence 'colorectal cancer' [CRC] in medical jargon) is the world's third most common cancer, accounting for about 10% of all cancers worldwide. Almost all medical authorities agree that alcohol is a major cause. For example, the WCRF says that there is "strong, convincing" evidence that drinking more than 30 grams of alcohol a day (roughly a third of a bottle of wine) will increase your risk of this often fatal cancer.

But what nobody (least of all the WCRF) tells you is that lower intakes of alcohol can actually *reduce* the risk. This extraordinary fact was pointed out in a recent large-scale review of the existing evidence in 2020.[33] Intakes of about 14 grams of alcohol a day were found to reduce CRC by a substantial 45%, and only at intakes of 56 grams did an increased risk of CRC begin to kick in. Even then, the extra risk was small: 20% at 98 grams a day.

There's a lot to take in here. For a start, what are alcohol grams? They are the amount of actual alcohol within a drink...any drink. For example, a standard bottle of wine contains 75 to 85 grams of alcohol, a pint of beer 20 grams, and a standard (70cl) bottle of spirits 224 grams.

Next, what about the extra risk percentage? On the face of it, it appears that 98 grams of alcohol (a bit more than is in a bottle of wine) will increase your cancer risk by 20%. If you're not mathematically-minded, that sounds like bad news, but it isn't. Why not?

Take the example of esophageal cancer at the start of this chapter, where Italian scientists found that drinking two bottles of wine a day increased risk by 18 times. Expressed in percentage terms, that's 1700% - yes, one thousand seven hundred percent.

Therefore, a 20% increased risk of anything is tiny - it's nowhere near even double the risk, which would be 100%. So in the grand scheme of things, 20% isn't really worth worrying about.

An everyday example amply proves the point.

One major study has demonstrated that if you simply add two spoonfuls of sugar to your daily tea or coffee, your extra risk of CRC rises by 50%, i.e. much less than double[34] - which is why you've never been warned about sugar and cancer. Sugar and obesity or diabetes, yes... but never cancer. That's because less than double the extra risk of anything is trivial.

And when we come to the wine evidence, the already tiny CRC risk not only disappears but does something extraordinary: it reverses.

Take a 2011 study by CRC experts in North Carolina. This was a massive undertaking, involving checking the health records of about a quarter of the state's population. The results were astonishing: first, only hard liquor drinkers were found to have an increased risk of the cancer; second, people who drank a modest amount of wine a day had a 30% decreased risk, and zero extra cancer risk at higher intakes.[35]

This was no fluke; there have been about half-a-dozen studies all pointing the same way.

In 2009 for example, Cambridge University researchers published the results of an 11-year study of almost 25,000 Britons, tracking their alcohol intake and risk of CRC. They too found that wine-drinkers had much less cancer than non-drinkers:

> Daily consumption of more than 8 grams of wine appeared inversely related to colorectal cancer risk (HR: 0.61).[36]

In plain English, wine drinkers were found to have almost half the bowel cancer risk of non-drinkers.

What's the secret of wine's medicinal powers in the gut? A clue has come from experiments by doctors at Spain's Laboratorio de Investigaciones Biomedicas. They gave male volunteers two glasses of red wine every day for 4 weeks, and found a marked increase in a range of beneficial bowel bacteria, and a corresponding reduction in pathogenic ones. "[This] suggests possible prebiotic benefits associated with the inclusion of red wine in the diet", they reported.[37]

So that could be the explanation: as we'll see in chapter 8, wine creates a healthy bacterial environment in the gut, thus discouraging the growth of one of our most common cancers.

However, the international data are "inconsistent", so the dull upshot is that the CRC/wine connection is overall neutral.[38]

Prostate Cancer

An unpleasant and really common cancer of men's old age: above the age of 65, it's a 50/50 toss-up whether you'll be diagnosed with it before you die.[39] For years, it's been believed that there is no food, drink or lifestyle way of preventing it, but a couple of decades ago the prestigious Fred Hutchinson Cancer Research Center in Seattle decided to give wine a chance to show its mettle. Astonishingly, their long-term study of 750 wine drinkers found that:

> Each additional glass of red wine consumed per week showed a statistically significant 6% decrease in relative risk of prostate cancer, with evidence for a decline in risk estimates across increasing categories of red wine intake. The more clinically aggressive prostate cancer is where the strongest reduction in risk was observed, (with a) 60% reduction in risk.[40]

In other words, the more wine the merrier – and particularly in the worst cases of the disease.

That sounds like very good news for men, but hold the celebrations: very few studies show such dramatic results, and indeed some show the reverse. In fact, a 2018 meta-analysis of the entire evidence base concludes that red wine has only a modest protective effect, and white wine the opposite. But the two wine figures are very low, leading the team of international researchers to conclude simply that "wine is not associated with an increased risk of prostate cancer."[41]

In other words, if you're a wine-tippling fella, don't worry – your risk of prostate cancer is still the same as everyone else's.

However, on the upside, wine really comes into its own if you actually succumb to prostate cancer. In 2019 Harvard researchers reported something remarkable: that men already diagnosed with prostate cancer halve their risk of dying from the disease if they drink wine after hearing the bad news...or in researcher-speak:

> Moderate red wine intake was associated with a lower risk (HR 0.50) of progression to lethal prostate cancer.[42]

What's "moderate"? Up to about a third of a bottle of wine a day, says Harvard. So, if you're unlucky to be diagnosed with prostate cancer, wine seem to be as good a 'medication' as the best pharmaceutical drugs around, and with none of the emasculating side-effects.

How wine performs such a miracle is a bit of a mystery. The nearest to an explanation comes from laboratory experiments where the constituents of red wine have been found to "inhibit" prostate cancer cells[43] and even prevent prostate cancer in mice.[44]

Lung cancer

By contrast, perhaps surprisingly, this is one cancer where wine really shines, particularly if you're an ex-smoker.

15

In a study on 84,170 American men, researchers at the Kaiser Permanente Research group in Pasadena found that, for each glass of red wine consumed per month, the risk of lung cancer declined by 2%. The most benefit – a staggering 85% reduction in risk – occurred in ex-smokers drinking more than a glass of wine a day.[45]

That research was reported in 2008, since when over twenty similar studies have been done, with broadly the same results. Wine drinkers have a significant decrease in lung cancer risk – even current smokers.[46]

There are no pharmaceutical drugs that can perform such magic, so what's so special about wine?

One small clue comes from Germany where 20 volunteers took part in an unusual clinical trial in 2017. They were made to smoke three Gauloises cigarettes preceded by a few hefty glasses of red wine (Chateau Haut-Pontet, Saint-Emilion Grand Cru 2005, no less!) The University of Saarland researchers reported finding that wine prevented tobacco's ill-effects on blood vessels:

> Endothelial damage, inflammation and cellular ageing were completely attenuated by red wine consumption..... (demonstrating) the potential of red wine as a protective strategy to avert markers of vascular injury.[47]

Stomach Cancer

Yet another good news story for wine, say top Danish researchers. Over a 28 year period, Professor Morten Grønbaek and his team at Copenhagen University tracked the drinking habits of nearly 30,000 people to check their stomach cancer ('gastric cancer' in medspeak) rates, and found that wine was hugely protective. The higher the intake, the more the prevention: a bottle of wine a week resulted in a 24% reduction in risk, but drinking more than two bottles a week produced a staggering 84% reduction – thus almost entirely abolishing the risk of stomach cancer. The Danes added that:

Linear trend test showed a significant association with a relative
risk ratio of 0.60 per glass of wine drunk per day.[48]

In other words, they found that every single glass of wine you drink a day reduces the risk of stomach cancer by 40%. There's no drug, vitamin pill or diet that can even approach that level of benefit.

But once again, there's disagreement among studies. In fact, the evidence overall is boringly neutral. A 2017 meta-analysis reports that wine has no effect one way or the other.[49] So the Danes might be a lucky special case.

Pancreatic Cancer

Although relatively uncommon, cancer of the pancreas is one of the most difficult to treat and is often rapidly fatal. It's also on the increase. There's some evidence that alcohol can be a risk factor, but mainly for spirits drinkers who also smoke.[50]

The real problem with alcohol is that it can cause the pancreas to become badly inflamed (pancreatitis), but you've got to be a seriously heavy drinker to succumb. The evidence is that:

Generally the onset of alcoholic pancreatitis occurs in the fourth
decade of males with an average alcohol consumption around
150 grams a day for a period of 10-15 years.[51]

At that intake level (a couple of bottles of wine a day for over a decade), wine appears to be just as harmful as any other booze. However, once again, folate supplements can come to the rescue, halving the cancer risk.[52]

Breast Cancer

I've left this highly emotive cancer till last, as it's the one which the medical authorities often use to strike fear in female drinkers - and by proxy, all drinkers. For example, official bodies such as the American Cancer Society routinely issue stern warnings such as:

> Alcohol increases risk of breast cancer. Even drinking small amounts of alcohol has been linked with an increase in risk. It is best not to drink alcohol at all.[53]

Here's a similar blast from the World Health Organisation:

> Alcohol consumption is one of the major modifiable risk factors, causing 7 of every 100 new breast cancer cases in Europe. There is no safe level of alcohol consumption.[54]

Sounds damning, as it's doubtless meant to. However, the evidence for a booze/breast cancer connection is not that clear-cut, with many uncertainties and outright contradictions in the evidence. For example, a 2019 study on about half a million Britons, although powerful enough to confirm drinkers' extra risk of esophageal cancer, found "no evidence of a causal association between alcohol consumption and breast cancer", despite using a variety of sophisticated statistical techniques.[55]

What about wine in particular? Here the evidence is clearer than with other booze types, with a surprising amount of good news for female drinkers.

Let's start with the home of wine - la Belle France, and in particular the Hérault Region "where wine is an integral part of the population's dietary habits", say two top French biostaticians, Professors Faiza Bessaoud and Jean-Pierre Daurès. Both senior scientists in INSERM (the equivalent of Britain's MRC or the US NIH), they did a massive two-year study to check out the alcohol/breast cancer issue. The procedure was simple: they identified every woman – young and old – who had been diagnosed with breast cancer. These women's entire lifestyles were then analysed in detail, including the types of alcohol they drank, how much and how often. There was another 'control group' of women without breast cancer for comparison.

The findings were dramatic. First, precisely echoing the sophisticated 2019 British study, none of the breast cancer cases appeared to have any association with alcohol intake – no matter how much nor what type of alcohol the women drank. Second, up to an intake of 15 grams of alcohol a day, wine *reduced the risk* of breast cancer – by a remarkable 42%, thus almost halving the cancer risk. Third, the greatest protection occurred among the women who drank wine every day; there was no benefit whatever if their intake was "sporadic". Fourth, higher intakes of wine did not increase cancer risk at all.

So the French experts had no option but politely to stick two fingers up to their quasi-prohibitionist (generally Anglophone) fellow researchers and declare that:

> Low and regular consumption of wine reduces the risk of breast cancer. This protective effect is due substantially to wine consumption, since the proportion of regular wine drinkers is predominant in our study population. It is (therefore) perhaps not suitable to advise that all low alcohol consumers, especially wine drinkers, reduce their alcohol intake.[56]

A 2014 population study on Greek women came to precisely the same conclusion, reporting that

> Moderate alcohol intake, and especially wine consumption, seems to be associated with breast cancer prevention.[57]

Fair enough, but we all know that the French and Greeks are particularly healthy human beings, mainly because of their Mediterranean diet. So you could argue they're a special case – and they probably are. But American wine-lovers aren't far behind them in the breast cancer stakes.

In 2009, six USA cancer centres pooled over 14,000 breast cancer cases for a study conducted for the prestigious (and highly conservative) National Cancer Institute. To everyone's surprise, the wine drinkers were found to have zero extra risk of breast cancer:

> In this large, multi-center, population-based case control study…neither red nor white wine was related to breast cancer.[58]

said the NCI researchers. The even better news was that, as with the French, drinking a medium-sized glass of red wine a day was found to have a modest preventive effect against breast cancer.

Intrigued by this red wine benefit, researchers at the Cedars-Sinai Heart Institute in Los Angeles persuaded (presumably with little difficulty) a group of pre-menopausal women to have a few drinks in the name of science. 36 volunteers were randomized to drink a large glass of Chardonnay (white) every day for a month, and Cabernet Sauvignon (red) the next month - or vice versa. In return, all they had to do was donate a few vials of blood.

The researchers were looking for any differences in the women's estrogen levels, because that's the hormone most implicated in breast cancer.

Interesting result: red wine was found to reduce estrogen (and incidentally increase testosterone) levels. So here was a possible explanation for red wine's breast cancer benefits. But why not white? The main difference between the two liquids is that white is made from just grape juice, while red also consists of the products of crushed grape skins, stalks and seeds. Astonishingly, that messy grape detritus contains chemicals which appear to mimic Big Pharma's 'aromatase inhibitors', costly anti-estrogen drugs often prescribed for breast cancer prevention.

> (Our) data suggest that red wine is a nutritional aromatase inhibitor, and may explain the observation that red wine does not appear to increase breast cancer risk.[59]

say the LA researchers.

Wine's AI benefits have been dramatically confirmed in breast cancer tests on mice at Caltech's Beckman Institute.

When researchers fed compounds derived from red wine to mice genetically engineered to get hormone-related breast cancer, they were astonished to find that:

> Our red wine extract completely abrogated ... neoplastic changes in mammary tissue.

In other words, there was no sign of breast cancer anywhere, despite the mice being programmed to succumb to it. The scientists were so impressed by the results that they made this remarkable suggestion:

> Red wine or red wine extract may be a chemo-preventive diet supplement for postmenopausal women who have a high risk of breast cancer.[60]

What makes these 'wine prevents breast cancer' results even more credible are three pioneering US research studies. The first was published in 1998 by scientists at the prestigious Mayo Clinic, who made the remarkable discovery that red wine appears to have some very healthy effects on actual breast tissue. This was discovered by chance in a long-term dietary survey of about 1500 women who were also undergoing routine mammography (breast cancer diagnosis by X-Ray). One of the survey's breast checks involved measuring the density of the breasts, as this is a known risk factor for breast cancer: the denser the breast tissue, the greater risk of cancer – up to 5 times higher.[61]

The remarkable chance discovery was this: drinking wine can affect breast density. The two wine types had opposing effects, however. Red wine drinkers were found to have less dense breasts, while it was the opposite for white wine drinkers. The density differences weren't great, but the overall trend was in red wine's favour. "The association with red wine is especially interesting in the light of the favourable associations reported with red wine and other diseases", the researchers noted.

That 1998 Mayo Clinic study was replicated a decade later by researchers at the equally prestigious Columbia University,

New York. While they found that drinkers in general had a modest (12%) increase in breast density, red wine drinkers' breasts were the reverse, with an up to 10% decrease. "We observed a consistent inverse association for red wine intake and mammographic density," reported the researchers. [62]

These very reassuring findings about the breast cancer risks of wine drinking will doubtless come as a huge surprise to my female readers, largely because they have never been reported in the mainstream media. Why? Clearly, the main reason is that they conflict with official dogma, but there's also a more understandable one: not all studies agree.

To date, there have been about 300 separate wine/breast cancer studies - some reassuring to drinkers, others not - so it's easy to select those which support any viewpoint. However, science has a way of arbitrating between disparate findings by the simple method of averaging them out, and trying to discern a pattern.

The technique is called meta-analysis, and in 2016 one such was conducted on the whole wine/breast cancer issue. Despite quite a lot of variability between the studies, after the data were pooled together, a conclusion was reached. Fortunately for wine drinkers, the evidence outlined above was confirmed, in that an anti-breast cancer effect was found – but only up to a relatively low wine intake.[63]

Here's a graph of the findings:

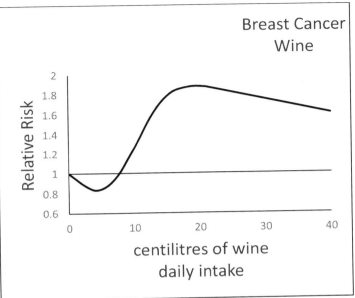

Derived from Chen J-Y et al (2016) "Dose-Dependent Associations between Wine Drinking and Breast Cancer Risk-Meta-Analysis Findings."Asian Pac J Cancer Prev 17.3: 1221-1233

The centre line (at 1.0) shows breast cancer risk among teetotallers, the wavy data line the risk among wine drinkers. The comparison demonstrates that the greatest protection against breast cancer occurs at a very low intake of about 5 centilitres of wine a day. But that soon falls away, with zero protection at 8 centilitres, rising to a 90% (i.e slightly less than double) increase in breast cancer risk at about a standard 15 cl glass. Note, however, that above that intake the risk declines - even at an intake of half a bottle of wine a day (37.5 cls).

That last finding raises an important question. Why is there a decline in risk when drinking more than a standard glass a day? Surely, if wine drinking really were a cause of breast cancer, one would expect a 'dose response': i.e. the higher the wine intake, the greater the cancer risk. But there isn't. That very fact brings up the whole issue of deciding between causality and correlation: how to establish whether something which merely appears to be connected to something else really is caused by it.

Fortunately, we can invoke the wisdom of Sir Austin Bradford Hill, the British medical statistician widely acknowledged as the major authority on the issue. Many years ago, he established nine principles of how to decide between a spurious correlation and a real causal link.[64] One of the most important was "biological gradient": a rise in health risk must mirror a rise in the putative cause; if it doesn't, he ruled, a causal link is unlikely. Another of his principles was "strength of association": if there was less than double the risk of extra harm, its causality was irrelevant. As is evident from the above graph, neither of those causality principles is satisfied on the wine/breast cancer issue.

The causality issue is further complicated by the fact that nobody has much of a clue how booze can cause cancer in the first place. Mouth, throat and gullet cancers are explicable [65], but it's hard to maintain for all the other ones, breast cancer included.

Why?

Because, once alcohol has got past the gullet and into the stomach and liver, the body's detoxifying toolkit of enzymes grabs hold of as much alcohol as it can manage, and processes it. First it converts alcohol to supposedly carcinogenic acetaldehyde, but almost as soon as that occurs, the toolkit doesn't allow acetaldehyde to persist, and "rapidly" reprocesses it into acetate.[66]

What's acetate? Also known as acetic acid, common examples are lemon juice and vinegar - totally harmless and certainly not carcinogenic.

In short, the body doesn't allow acetaldehyde to hang around long enough to do any damage (although not among very heavy drinkers: see the FAQ chapter at the end of this book). So there is currently no cogent explanation for alcohol causing the vast majority of cancers.

But back to wine and breast cancer.

I recognise that women may be sceptical about the 'good news' research I've cited - and understandably after the scare stories they've been subjected to over the years. Furthermore, even taking the figures on the graph above at face value, women should compare them to the hazards of drinking another everyday liquid...milk. One study on over 50,000 Americans showed that drinking as little as 1.5 "cups" of milk a day is the equivalent of drinking half a bottle of wine a day in terms of the extra breast cancer risk.[67]

Another study on Chinese women found pretty much the same.[68]

Hmm.... so drinking milk is associated with some extra breast cancer risk.* But have you ever heard the medical authorities issue the same kinds of dire anti-milk warnings as they do with booze? Neither have I.

Folate Magic

But let's assume that there is a causal link - however small - between wine and breast cancer. What can worried women do about it? The good news is that, for those who overindulge (in any type of alcohol, not just wine) there's a very simple answer: the magic B vitamin, folate. A major study shows that if young women drinkers take a daily supplement of 400 mg of folate, they will reduce their extra breast cancer risk to almost zero - even those with a family history of breast cancer. Indeed, drinkers with no family history will *totally eliminate the extra breast cancer risk associated with alcohol.* Those astonishing discoveries were made in 2017 by a team of Harvard University epidemiologists in their celebrated Nurses' Health Study, one of medicine's longest-running health surveys.[69]

---

* The milk/breast cancer connection is much less than twice the extra risk, but if women milk drinkers are worried about what I've reported, they should switch to soy milk, which may actually have a small preventive effect, says the research study.

Similar findings have been made in post-menopausal women, although with less dramatic outcomes.[70] [71] What is clear, however, is that the magic only derives from folate, and not from its synthetic formulation, folic acid - indeed folic acid may actually be harmful for some people.[72]

Cancer: the Good News

This very long chapter finally ends with some very good news for drinkers, as there are half-a-dozen cancers which are actually *prevented* by alcohol – all types of booze, not just wine.

First, **kidney cancer,** the world's eighth most common cancer, whose incidence has been steadily increasing year by year, and now accounts for 3% of all cancers. But alcohol is in no way to blame – in fact, quite the reverse.

In 2007, scientists at Harvard University did a massive synthesis of all the existing research findings investigating the alcohol/kidney cancer link. Here's what they found:

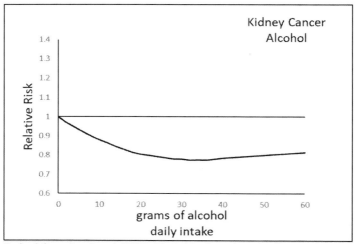

Derived from: Lee J et al (2007) Alcohol intake and renal cell cancer in a pooled analysis of 12 prospective studies. J Natl Cancer Inst. 99(10):801-10.

As is clear, kidney cancer risk decreases pretty consistently among drinkers – even up to a relatively high 60 grams a day. Why? The 27 experts on the Harvard team were puzzled. Could the nutrients in wine and beer have been responsible? No. The data showed that people who drank mainly spirits were also protected against kidney cancer – and spirits are neat alcohol plus water. The logic was inescapable. "The finding that all three types of alcoholic beverages were associated with lower risk suggests that alcohol *per se* is most likely the responsible factor," the researchers had to conclude.

But surely there must be a point at which high intakes of alcohol damage the kidneys? Apparently not, according to a later Italian study on heavy drinkers which had even more dramatic findings than the Harvard one, reporting:

> Risk of kidney cancer continued to decrease even above 100 grams/day of alcohol intake, with no apparent levelling in risk.[73]

In fact, the evidence as a whole says that your kidneys will welcome being dunked in any amount of alcohol...and of any type: wine, beer or spirits.[74]

Indeed, alcohol reduces your risk of all types of kidney problems [75], a finding confirmed in autopsies where pathologists have been amazed by the health of drinkers' kidneys.[76]

There's good news for your thyroid gland, too.

Although **thyroid cancer** is relatively uncommon, its incidence is rising inexorably, particularly in women. Drinking could "significantly" bring this rate down, according to the US National Cancer Institute. In a huge NCI study on about half a million people conducted over a period of 7½ years, the results were unequivocal:

> Compared with non-drinking, consuming two or more drinks per day was associated with a significantly decreased risk of thyroid cancer. The risk of thyroid cancer decreased with increasing

alcohol consumption by approximately 6 percent per 10 grams consumed daily.[77]

This isn't a freak finding: most studies have confirmed an anti-cancer effect.[78]

Even more surprising, given that alcohol's effects are primarily transmitted via the bloodstream, **blood cancers** are also significantly reduced among drinkers.

The first researchers to make this astonishing discovery were part of Iowa's Women's Health Study in the 1980s and 90s. Unexpectedly, women who drank more than a minuscule amount of alcohol a day (3.5 grams = a Budweiser) were found to reduce their risk of Non-Hodgkin Lymphoma (NHL) by almost 40%.[79]

Iowa's bizarre data kick-started an international scramble to confirm the findings…or more likely refute them ("a Bud preventing a major cancer? You cannot be serious!"). By 2005, four countries' experts had analysed 15,000 people's health records - and lo and behold, Iowa was vindicated: drinkers of all types of alcohol were found to have a 20% reduced risk of NHL, and a staggering 50% risk reduction of another type of blood cancer called Burkitt's Lymphoma.[80]

It was then the turn of the American Cancer Society to try and refute this evident nonsense. But when they checked the health records of over a million Americans, they too confirmed the Iowa data…with an unexpected twist: the heaviest drinkers had the most benefit:

Compared with non-drinkers, the relative risk of NHL reduced by 7% below 14 grams of alcohol a day, by 9% below 28 grams, and by 28% at higher intakes.[81]

But the most dramatic findings came in 2014 from Sweden, a country with a huge drinking problem. It also has a centralized health system with some very reliable national health records (known as the Swedish Registry), from which cancer experts identified over 420,000 people with "alcohol use disorders". The Registry revealed that, although these very heavy drinkers had more than double the risk of gullet and throat cancers (as you'd expect), they had major reductions in the risk of blood-borne cancers: leukemia (49% less), myeloma (48% less), NHL (35% less), and Hodgkin disease (29% less).

> Our data suggest that alcohol consumption has a protective effect against hematological malignancies (i.e. blood cancers)...[even for] people with severe alcohol consumption – a somewhat novel finding.[82]

reported the researchers wryly.

Multiple Myeloma is a "rare but highly fatal" cancer of the bone marrow, according to a team of international experts who in 2013, under the auspices of the National Cancer Institute, examined over 1500 cases of the disease, and found that teetotallers had nearly double the risk of the disease than drinkers.[83]

Women wine-drinkers are particularly protected against this cancer, according to a world-wide survey in 2015.[84]

Summary

Wine drinking and cancer is a very complicated picture, partly because the evidence for a connection is so contradictory: some studies say drinking increases the risk, others say the reverse.

Also, much depends on 1. how much wine you drink, 2. the type of cancer.

Heavy long-term wine drinking will increase the risk of cancers of the pancreas, mouth, throat and gullet, but moderate intake may reduce the risk of the last.

A minority of heavy wine drinkers are at risk of liver cirrhosis.

The Very Good News About Wine

Heavy wine drinking is associated with a marginal increase of the risk of cancers of the liver and possibly the breast.

Moderate wine drinking is associated with a decrease in the risk of cancers of the lung and, in some studies, of the breast.

Any level of wine intake will have no effect on stomach or bowel cancer risk, and some studies show it will reduce the risk.

Any level of alcohol intake will decrease the risk of cancers of the kidney, thyroid and blood.

The carcinogenic effects of all alcohols can be largely prevented by maintaining adequate levels of vitamin B9 (Folate) in the bloodstream.

3

Heart Disease

If the media ever reports any positive news about alcohol and health, heart disease is the one condition that always comes up as benefiting from drinking. And rightly so. For there are literally hundreds of separate studies conducted over the last 50 years, which overwhelmingly show that drinkers - of wine, in particular - have much less heart disease than teetotallers. Indeed, the evidence is so strong that, if wine had been invented in a laboratory, pharmaceutical companies would be selling it by the tanker-load as a super-powerful heart disease medication.

But of course, the reality is that wine is a natural substance and therefore can't be patented. What's more, much of the medical profession (plus a small coterie of anti-alcohol researchers) disapprove of alcohol *per se*, making it ideologically and politically impossible for them to acknowledge any health benefits.

Hence there's a tug of war – sometimes battled in the media - between the majority of experts who say wine is good heart medicine and a band of vocal opponents who deny it. But this is too important an issue to have ideological wars over. After all, heart disease is the world's Number One killer, and if something as simple as downing a few glasses of wine a day can 'cure' it, that could have a huge impact on global health.

So, what are the facts? Let's look at the actual data.

The Evidence

The first the world heard about the wine/heart disease story was in the 1980s, with headlines about the "French Paradox".

This was the term coined by two French Government scientists to explain why their compatriots had nearly half the heart disease of other countries (the USA in particular), despite the well-known Gallic love of foods high in saturated fat[85] – the kind of eating habits believed to be the major cause of heart disease. Anglophone nutritionists were mystified by the fact that the French weren't dropping dead like flies from their *foie gras, saucissons, fromages, croissants au beurre* etc. The explanation was that their equally high intake of wine must somehow be counteracting the "unhealthy" fats.

The discovery of the French Paradox not only dropped a bomb on the prevailing theory about fats and heart disease, but also kick-started a slew of alcohol/heart disease studies around the world. One of the first results had already come from Britain. Back in the 1950s, Oxford University scientists came up with the brilliant idea of persuading over 10,000 doctors to provide regularly updated details of their health status and lifestyles (food, alcohol, tobacco, exercise etc.), to see if there was any connection between the two. The Oxford experts' most famous discovery was the link between smoking and lung cancer. But arguably even more dramatic was their discovery of a link between heart disease and drinking.

Astonishingly, in complete contrast to those doctors who didn't smoke, the doctors who didn't drink were found to be the least healthy, in that they died earlier from heart disease. Indeed, the Oxford team found that non-drinkers had twice the death rates of men who drank even as much as the equivalent of a bottle of wine a day.[86]

Not to be outdone, the equally prestigious Harvard University joined in the fun. Their scientists also persuaded an even larger group of "health professionals" to send in regular detailed reports on their lifestyle and health status. Within 20 years, a clear pattern had emerged about alcohol intake and heart disease.

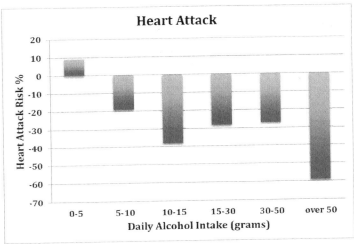

Derived from: Joline WJ et al 2007.Alcohol consumption and risk for coronary heart disease among men with hypertension *Ann Intern Med.* 2;146(1):10-9

This chart shows the frequency of heart attacks among the men who drank different daily amounts of alcohol; the zero line is non-drinkers' risk of heart attacks. As you can see, apart from those who drank tiny amounts of alcohol, the more these men drank the less their chance of a heart attack. Drinking 10 to 15 grams a day reduced risk by nearly 40%, and over 50 grams a day (= over half a bottle of wine) by nearly 60%.

Buoyed up by the Oxford and Harvard findings, other (mainly US) academics piled into heart disease/alcohol research, and confirmed that alcohol is good medicine not only for the heart but for the whole cardiovascular system – for example, halving of the risk of heart failure[87], high blood pressure[88] and ischemic stroke.[89]

European research groups, surveying their own national populations, also found that drinking has substantial benefits for cardiovascular health. However, everyone agreed that there was a stumbling block: above a certain alcohol intake, the 'medicine' stops working and becomes toxic.

By the beginning of this century, enough studies had been done to be able to pool the results in a meta-analysis, and the graph that emerged was a stark illustration of the alcohol/heart disease issue.

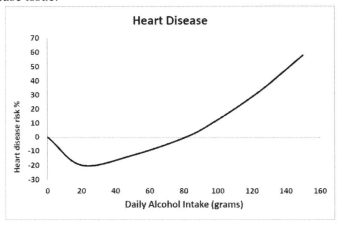

Adapted from: Corrao G et al Addiction. 2000 Oct;95(10):1505-23. Alcohol and coronary heart disease: a meta-analysis.

The zero line across the middle is the standard risk of heart disease among people who don't drink. The curved line traces the risk of heart disease among drinkers, according to how much they normally drink per day.

It shows that those who drink between 18 to 30 grams of alcohol a day reduce their risk of heart disease by about 20% compared to if they'd never touched a drop. It also shows that some kind of protective effect persists up to about 70 grams a day. Above this, the heart disease risk increases. This is what statisticians call a J-curve, because the graph of the data has that shape.

J-curves are not uncommon in other medical areas. Take sports medicine. It's now well established that athletes who train at moderate levels of exertion reduce their overall risks of ill-health, but the risks go into reverse if they "over-train".[90] Of course, the most famous example of 'the more not

34

necessarily the merrier' is plain water: drinking either none or a huge amount is equally fatal.*

But alcohol seems to be special in that it's a powerful heart disease preventive, and yet actually causes the very same disease at high doses. Why?

One reason may be that alcohol in quantity can trigger high blood pressure ('hypertension' in medspeak). This was first noticed during World War One when a French doctor observed that front-line soldiers who drank more than two litres of wine a day (yes, almost three bottles!) had four times the risk of hypertension compared to "sober" men drinking "only" a litre of wine a day.[91] By the way, the ration for French soldiers in the trenches was 2 litres of wine a day – then considered to be a "moderate" intake.

Hypertension puts a strain on the heart and blood vessels, and is therefore a logical risk factor for heart disease. Its most obvious consequence is hemorrhagic strokes – mini-explosions of blood in the brain. But oddly enough, as already mentioned, moderate drinking *prevents* another type of stroke: the ischemic stroke.[92]

How come? Well, ischemic strokes happen when blood is blocked from entering parts of the brain, often caused by blood clots. The theory is that alcohol thins the blood, thus preventing blockages. But even so, above an intake of 40 grams a day, the benefit goes gently into reverse.[93]

More alarming is the discovery that long-term heavy drinkers run the risk of atrial fibrillation (rapid irregular heart beat)[94], atherosclerosis (furred-up arteries) - possibly as bad as the risk from smoking, according to Austrian researchers[95] - and cardiomyopathy, a heart-wasting disease which ultimately ends in heart failure.[96]

These risks easily explain how high alcohol intakes send the heart health benefits at lower intakes into reverse – hence the J-curve.

---

* In fact, water intake and death is not a J-, but a U-curve

Backlash

You would have thought that all this negative information about the dangers of high intakes of alcohol would have been music to the ears of the medical profession, who have long advocated abstinence from alcohol on health grounds – despite, of course, many doctors not practising what they preached.

But no. They were up in arms about.that pesky beginning of the J-curve: the fact that at relatively low intakes, drinkers have less risk of heart disease than non-drinkers. It stuck in their craw that alcohol could possibly have any health benefits.

So they set about encouraging academics to cast doubt on the J-curve findings.

The first wrecking ball thrown at the J-curve was the idea that non-drinkers are not a valid comparison group to drinkers. This was the theory proposed by a team of researchers led by London University Professor A.G. Shaper who suggested that non-drinkers might already be suffering from various ailments, or more importantly were ex-drinkers who had become teetotal because alcohol made them ill. He called them "sick quitters".[97]

Suddenly, everyone realised Shaper could be right: if unwell ex-drinkers are included in the teetotal comparison groups, this will inevitably make drinkers appear to be relatively healthier.[98]

So, many alcohol/heart disease researchers scuttled back to their original data, weeding out all the non-drinkers who might have been sick quitters. They then re-analysed their data, thus making a genuine comparison between drinkers and 100% healthy teetotallers.

What effect did this have on their original findings?

As it turned out, not much. Although there were slight reductions in the apparent heart health benefits of alcohol, they weren't nearly large enough to nullify the basic J-curve.

For example, when Professor Eric Rimm and his Harvard colleagues went back to the medical data on their "51,529 male health professionals" and removed everyone who could conceivably have been a sick quitter, this still "did not substantially affect the relative risks," they reported, adding that they felt the case was now closed, declaring that:

> These findings support the hypothesis that the inverse relation between alcohol consumption and risk of coronary disease is causal.[99]

In other words, drinking really does help prevent heart disease.

To double-check they were right, the same Harvard team picked out nearly 9000 people from the pool of health professionals, chosen because they and their lifestyles were exceptionally healthy – i.e. not a single sicko among them. Most of them were drinkers, and about a quarter were teetotallers. They were then all closely monitored for 16 years, during which it was found that most heart attacks occurred among the non-drinkers.[100]

Interestingly, Harvard also found that, in contrast to current medical advice to abstain from alcohol for at least two days a week, the evidence suggests that it's regular daily drinking that confers the greatest protection against heart disease:

> An intake of 30 grams of alcohol a day [has] an overall predicted 24.7% reduction in risk of coronary heart disease. [101]

Faced with this mass of evidence pointing one way, all but a handful of die-hard sceptics now regard the sick quitter theory as itself a sick and indeed rather dead duck. If you're in any doubt about this, these are the references to just some of the relevant studies:[102 103 104 105 106 107 108 109 110 111 112 113]

Bodily evidence

The most compelling reason to be so confident about the fact that booze is good news for hearts comes from drinkers' actual bodies. Let's start with their arteries.

Furred-up arteries (atherosclerosis in medspeak) are a major cause of heart disease, and moderate drinkers have fairly consistently been shown to have less furry ones. The easiest way to check on someone's arteries is with ultrasound. One study using this technique found that moderate drinkers (up to 50 grams a day) had half the atherosclerosis of non-drinkers.[114] Alcohol is also a boon if you like to eat artery-clogging transfats, because drinking significantly protects you against the associated risk of atherosclerosis.[115]

Next, drinkers' blood.

When researchers have given people alcohol under laboratory test conditions, some dramatic things occur in their bloodstreams, the most important of which is a significant increase in levels of 'high-density lipoprotein cholesterol', otherwise known as HDL. It's commonly called the 'good' cholesterol as high HDL levels are known to protect against heart disease.[116]

Harvard experts have analysed the results of over 40 laboratory trials on human volunteers, and found that ingesting alcohol significantly raises HDL levels – far more effectively than the best drugs available. They reported finding that:

> Alcohol consumption increased HDL cholesterol levels by about 0.1 mmol/L overall and in a dose-response manner.... This degree of increase is greater than any currently available single pharmacological therapy.[117]

Human guinea-pig trials have also confirmed alcohol's value as a blood-thinner, helping to explain why it helps prevent ischemic strokes.[118]

Laboratory tests also show it reduces the so-called 'inflammatory markers' of heart disease, such as C-reactive protein, fibrinogen and homocysteine.[119]

These clinical observations are not one-offs: they have been repeatedly found in laboratories across the world[120], offering a strong scientific rationale for alcohol's health benefits. Summarising the evidence, Harvard Professor Eric Rimm concluded:

The combined beneficial effect of alcohol on the underlying biological mechanisms...can almost entirely explain the reduced heart disease risk among moderate drinkers.[121]

More Backlash

Once again, you might have thought that the medical profession would welcome such a breakthrough. After all, it's precisely the kind of supporting clinical evidence required of the pharmaceutical industry in marketing its drugs. With alcohol in moderation now firmly established as one answer to the world's No 1 killer, you'd have expected the authorities to be delighted that drinkers were unwittingly reducing their risk of heart disease.

But no. Yet more sceptical academics were recruited to muddy the waters. Having failed to win the "sick quitter" argument, they then turned to genetics to claim that the whole idea that drinkers have less heart disease is complete phooey.

I won't bore you with the details, as the 'genetics analyses' (called Mendelian Randomisation) are complex, and in any case have failed to produce clear-cut results. Also, many of these studies have been conducted on Asians who lack the necessary alcohol-detoxifying enzymes (see chapter 6), and therefore have limited relevance for the majority of drinkers. What's more, introducing genetics heavily restricts the size of the studies, so it's difficult to get 'statistically significant' findings, explaining why the genetic analysis technique is becoming almost as much a dead duck as the sick quitter hypothesis,[122] [123] except in the minds of a handful of diehard sceptics.

Back to wine

In any case, this research has been about all types of alcohol. What about wine? Is it any better for your heart than straight alcohol? Until the end of the turn of the century, the answer was no: beer, wine and spirits are equally valuable in heart disease, people thought.[124]

But that view has now begun to change: wine turns out to be even better.

That breakthrough discovery about wine's extra heart health benefits has largely come from Spain. In the early part of this century, doctors at the University of Barcelona's Institut d'Investigacions Biomèdiques embarked on a major alcohol research programme, treating wine like a new experimental drug, and testing its effects on healthy men in laboratory conditions. They used the standard technique for comparing the efficacy of two rival pharmaceutical drugs: a 'randomised crossover' experimental design – 4 weeks taking drug one, and 4 weeks taking drug two. Here, the two comparison drugs were wine (a few glasses per day) versus gin (a few measures a day). The amounts of alcohol in each case were the same: 30 grams.

What the Spanish researchers were looking for were changes in the body's 'biomarkers' for heart disease. Here are some examples of what they found:

Red wine:

1. Reduces "inflammatory biomarkers of atherosclerosis"; in other words, it helps stop the body producing some of the substances that cause furred-up arteries. Gin is pretty good too, but red wine is even better.[125]

2. Improves "glucose metabolism and the lipid profile, conferring protective effects on cardiovascular disease". Both gin and red wine increase HDL ('good' cholesterol) and healthy lipoproteins, but only red wine seems to decrease insulin levels - an extra plus for diabetes prevention.[126]

3. "Decreases erythrocyte superoxide dismutase (SOD) activity." SOD is bad news for heart disease as it increases blood oxidation, creating harmful blood contents such as LDL ('bad') cholesterol. Red wine significantly counteracts this effect, thus making it a useful antioxidant. Gin is not nearly as good.[127]

4. Nearly abolishes "monocyte adhesion", thus helping to reduce atherosclerosis - and again much better than gin.[128]

Spanish women were also tested – although they received less booze than the men (20 grams of alcohol a day). Their human guinea-pig role was to see if white as well as red wine might benefit heart disease's "inflammatory biomarkers". The results clearly showed that both wine types significantly reduce many of these heart disease precursors, but that red is more powerful.[129]

All these tests of alcohol's effects on people's bodies are unequivocal evidence that both alcohol itself and wine in particular have major effects on the biochemistry of heart disease. These are immensely important findings, because the clinical trial design used by the Spanish researchers is incontestable evidence-based medicine – you can't get any better proof than that.

There are two major implications.

First, the controversies about the epidemiological evidence for alcohol's benefits in heart disease can be set aside. It can no longer be legitimate to argue that these are imaginary, caused by artefacts such as "sick quitters" or other "confounders". The mechanisms of how alcohol prevents heart disease are now established by hard laboratory data, turning mere correlation into real causation.

Indeed, the evidence for alcohol's heart benefits is so strong that it has close to the status of scientific proof, summed up here by Professor Jorgen Rehm of Toronto University, one of the world's most respected alcohol researchers.

> For drinkers having one to two drinks per drinking day... there is substantial and consistent evidence from epidemiological and short-term experimental studies for a beneficial association with heart disease risk when compared to lifetime abstainers. The alcohol-heart disease relationship fulfills all criteria for a causal association.[130]

The clinical studies' other implication is that, although alcohol (in moderation) has major heart disease benefits, wine is better still.

Two studies from wine-drinking countries amply prove the point.

At the turn of this century, the French government did a "National Epidemiologic Survey on Alcohol and Related Conditions" involving a cross-section of the drinking population. Being France, many of the drinkers were fairly heavy boozers, with over 20% of them classified as "hazardous drinkers" - and a goodly number outright alcoholics. To everyone's surprise – possibly not least to the alcoholics themselves - the medical authorities reported that they all had a substantially reduced risk of heart disease, with the greatest reduction among the heaviest drinkers.

> Our study shows that alcohol may have cardio-protective effects (i.e. heart disease benefits) not only in moderate drinkers but also in individuals with patterns of use traditionally considered as hazardous.[131]

It was the same story in Spain where a ten-year study came up with almost identical findings: "moderate" wine drinkers were found to reduce their risk of heart disease by about 35%, but "very high consumers" had an even greater drop in risk, at 50%. Unlike other alcohol types, there was no J-curve, nor even a U-curve, but a straight line correlation. More wine, less heart disease.[132]

However, as is common in epidemiology, not all studies agree. When they're all pooled together, this is what emerges:

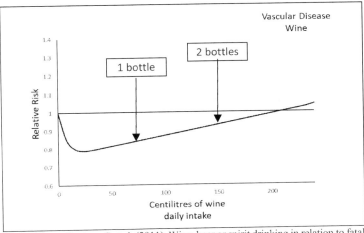

Derived from: Costanz, S et al. (2011). Wine, beer or spirit drinking in relation to fatal and non-fatal cardiovascular events: a meta-analysis. *European journal of epidemiology*, 26(11), 833-850.

This meta-analysis was done in 2011 by a group of Italian biologists widely acknowledged as some of the leading experts in alcohol research. Their graph clearly shows the beneficial effect of wine on the risk of both getting and dying from vascular disease, a major cause of heart problems. Once again, the evidence comes out as a J-shaped curve, with 25% maximal risk reduction at about 30 centilitres of wine a day and significant protection continuing up to a bottle of wine a day. However, although the graph shows some benefit persisting above that intake level, the Italian group cautions against taking it too literally, as the evidence is more uncertain at higher intakes.

In any case, what is abundantly clear is that wine is overwhelmingly the best alcohol type for heart disease prevention. Compare the 'wine graph' above with the 'alcohol graph' on page 34. Wine's J-curve is much flatter, meaning it's more beneficial than alcohol itself.

Furthermore, wine appears to be much more effective than the panoply of medications commonly prescribed for heart disease prevention – Ace Inhibitors, Angiotensin Receptor

Blockers, Anticoagulants, Antiplatelet agents, Statins, Digitalis, Diuretics, Vasodilators etc. – and, of course, far more enjoyable to ingest.

Indeed, if you're already at risk of heart disease, wine could arguably be the medication of choice, say French doctors. Take the case of essential hypertension (chronic high blood pressure), a known risk factor for heart disease and premature death. In a 20-year study on over 35,000 hypertensive blue-collar workers, the researchers found that men who drank up to a bottle of wine a day "had significantly lower risks of death by (up to) 37% than did abstainers."[133]

How does wine become such powerful medicine? Here are three examples among many, discovered in yet more clinical trials: wine clears the arteries of harmful fats after heart attacks[134]; it reduces blood levels of homocysteine, a major destroyer of arteries[135]; and it boosts blood levels of Omega-3 fatty acids.[136]

This last is particularly important, because Western diets are often deficient in Omega-3s, increasing the risk of heart disease.[137]

Summary

Heart disease is the world's No, 1 killer, but teetotallers are more at risk than drinkers, particularly wine drinkers.

Sceptics claim this evidence is phoney, but clinical trials testing wine like a pharmaceutical drug demonstrate how and why it is of benefit at moderate daily intakes.

4

Diabetes

Once fairly rare, Type 2 diabetes is one of the fastest-growing health problems in the world – indeed it's now at "epidemic proportions". According to the WHO, it now has over 400 million victims worldwide – up from about 100 million in the 1980s.

It's particularly rife in countries dominated by Big Food, such as the USA and Britain. It's hugely debilitating, causing major curtailments to sufferers' quality of life, as well as more severe problems such as heart attacks, blindness, and even leg amputations.

It's also expensive to treat: Big Pharma reckons it will be a $60 billion business in 2025 - all paid for by Joe Public, of course.

Wouldn't it be nice if international health providers could halt this tidal wave of diabetes cheaply and easily?

Well, they can…but how?

You've guessed it, of course: it's by prescribing alcohol.

There have been over 2000 studies on the diabetes/alcohol link. The latest meta-analysis of the highest quality research studies shows startling evidence that moderate drinkers have a substantially reduced risk of getting diabetes.[138]

Here's a graph of the dramatic evidence:

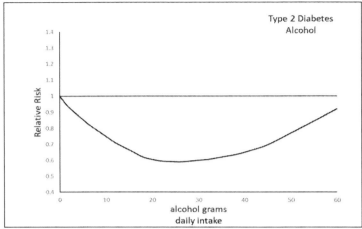

Derived from Li XH et al (2016). Association between alcohol consumption and the risk of incident type 2 diabetes: a systematic review and dose-response meta-analysis. *The American journal of clinical nutrition*, 103(3), 818-829].

The graph shows a robust (about 25%) reduced risk of diabetes occurring at an intake of 20 to 30 grams of alcohol a day, and that even double that intake will still offer some protection.

In other words, the evidence shows that a major risk factor for diabetes is abstaining from alcohol.

But binge drinking is a no-no, says another international survey:

> [Although] long-term alcohol use is associated with improved glycemic control....and reduces the incidence of diabetes, binge drinking seems to increase the incidence.[139]

What about wine itself? Well, a 2017 study of nearly half a million people showed that it's more effective than beer and spirits, with the most diabetes protection occurring at an intake of about a third of a bottle of wine a day, in a similar graph to the one above.[140]

But how does alcohol work such magic?

Glucose, Insulin etc.

As is well known, Type 2 diabetes is an excess of glucose (mainly derived from carbohydrate foods) in the bloodstream, generally triggered by a failure of the body to respond to insulin, the hormone that regulates glucose levels.

What is less well known is that alcohol has some unique effects on this whole process, by causing the human body "significantly" to reduce its production of glucose.[141]

How does alcohol do that? Answer: by reducing insulin levels.

Low insulin levels are generally a very healthy sign, and far more desirable than the opposite.

High insulin levels are associated with weight gain, high blood pressure, increased LDL (bad) cholesterol, inflammation of the arteries, heart disease, cancer – and, of course, diabetes. Why? Because high insulin is a sign of 'insulin resistance', indicating that the glucose regulation system isn't running efficiently, and the body has to pump more insulin into the system to force it to work properly.

This is not controversial. Health authorities across the world recommend reducing insulin levels in order to reduce your risk of diabetes and other nasties. Doctors recommend a variety of solutions: do more exercise, reduce your weight, and take loads of pharmaceuticals (natch). But nowhere do they say 'drink alcohol'.

And yet take a look at this chart.

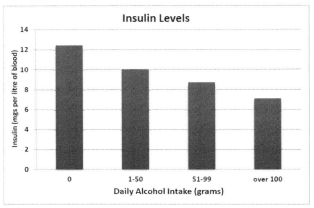

Derived from: Kiechl S et al. Insulin sensitivity and regular alcohol consumption: large prospective, cross-sectional population study BMJ, 1996, 313, 1040-1044

It comes from a clinical study testing the insulin levels in the blood of of nearly one thousand predominantly wine-drinking Italians – some drinking way over a bottle a day.

What's immediately striking is the fact that the higher the alcohol intake, the lower the insulin levels. It's a perfect 'dose response', strongly indicating that alcohol itself is the cause of this healthy reduction in insulin.[142]

That evidence was published in the prestigious BMJ in 1996, meaning 1. no-one could have missed it, and 2. it's been known for over a quarter of a century. Ten years later, much more work had been done on the subject, reinforcing the Italian data:

> The results of published studies on alcohol consumption and type 2 diabetes consistently indicate that moderate alcohol consumption reduces the risk of type 2 diabetes. The risk reduction is in the order of 30%, comparable to what has been reported for cardiovascular disease. A protective effect of moderate alcohol consumption is compatible with findings that alcohol can enhance insulin sensitivity. Whether high alcohol intake actually increases the risk of type 2 diabetes is unclear.[143]

And yet such clear evidence has been consistently ignored by diabetes doctors. Although alcohol is probably the most effective reducer of insulin levels, it's still not recommended to prevent diabetes.

Alcohol as Diabetes Therapy

Next question: what if you're in danger of getting diabetes or have already got it? Can alcohol help? There's some evidence it might.

For example, in 2004 an international group of researchers tested people with already established 'insulin resistance' (a pre-diabetic condition) and found that 40 grams of alcohol a day reduced the resistance problem by over 20%.[144]

Another group of people at high risk of diabetes are kidney transplant recipients. Traditionally, they've been told to lay off the booze, but it's now clear that the abstinence instruction was hogwash, and doubtless hastened the deaths of many thousands of transplantees. For in 2010 doctors at Groningen University Medical Centre in Holland discovered that transplantees who ignored medical advice and regularly drank "moderate" amounts of alcohol reduced their diabetes risk by 67%, and premature death by a substantial 44%.[145]

What about alcohol helping people who've already got full-blown diabetes? Sadly, very few research scientists have addressed this question. That's hardly surprising, as the advice doled out to diabetics is to avoid the demon drink, possibly because getting tipsy might make them forget about their special diet.

However, such nannying advice has often been ignored by diabetics. Indirectly, this disobedient "up yours, doc" attitude has been a gift to science, because it has enabled researchers to check whether official advice to diabetics to lay off the booze is evidence-based or not.

Well, it isn't. Here's the story.

In about 2008, doctors began tracking over 10,000 diabetics across twenty countries, monitoring their alcohol intake and general health. Five years later, the medics compared the obedient non-drinkers with the disobedient drinkers - the "goody-goodies" versus the "up-yours", if you like. You can probably guess who won. On average the goody-goodies had roughly a 20% greater risk of heart disease – and indeed premature death - than the up-yours. But of course there was a limit: heavy-drinking diabetics ended up as badly off as the goody-goodies. The ideal intake was found to be up to about 30 grams of alcohol a day (= a third of a bottle of wine). By the way, wine drinkers again came out the clear winners.[146]

In another study, when diabetics drank half a bottle of red wine a day for just two weeks,

> whole body glucose disposal improved by 43%... markedly attenuat(ing) insulin-resistance.[147]

So the totality of the wine/alcohol and diabetes evidence is a yet another good news story to add to the heart disease findings. In fact, it's no coincidence that alcohol helps both conditions, because they are closely connected: diabetics have up to four times greater risk of dying of heart disease.

Another close relative of diabetes is:

Metabolic Syndrome

This condition is increasingly in the news because it's a rapidly growing problem, especially in the USA. Although uncommon half a century ago, it now afflicts about 1 in 3 Americans – young women in particular.[148]

Strictly speaking, Metabolic Syndrome (*aka* Syndrome X) isn't a disease but a collection of health problems which appear to be unrelated, but often occur simultaneously. The typical victim is obese, with a large waist size, high blood pressure, an unhealthy cholesterol ratio, and incipient diabetes.

Drinking can substantially reduce the risk of developing this life-shortening condition, according to a summary of international studies, which found that:

> Alcohol consumption of less than 40 grams/day in men and 20 grams/day in women significantly reduced the prevalence of metabolic syndrome. [149]

Red wine can be even more beneficial, reducing metabolic syndrome biomarkers by as much as 70%, Israeli researchers reported in 2015 after a two year clinical trial. How much wine do you need to achieve such a dramatic effect? Just a small glass every day with an evening meal.[150]

Yet again, why is a glass of wine - simple, cheap and happily consumed with food the world over - never recommended to prevent this grisly condition?

Summary

Diabetes is a huge global problem, but alcohol can come to the rescue, significantly reducing its risk among drinkers. Wine is particularly beneficial, even in Metabolic Syndrome, one of today's more intractable conditions.

5

Dementia

Dementia has been chillingly described as robbing people of every faculty that makes them human. It's almost exclusively a disease of old age, and now that life expectancy has risen dramatically (apart from the recent Covid-related blip), more of us are living long enough to be at risk of succumbing to it. It can also be a very drawn-out disease. My own mother, despite having had a successful career as a high-powered mathematician, succumbed in her eighties, and took almost a decade to die from it.

What could have saved her and the millions of people whom the disease kills every year?

Despite the occasional over-hyped "breakthroughs" reported in the media, there are no cures for it. So what else is there? Could wine come to the rescue?

The first people to investigate whether different types of alcohol might help in this appalling disease were the Swedes. Way back in 1968, they began a medical monitoring job which lasted 34 years. The study group was made up of 1500 middle-aged women whose drinking habits were noted over the years. The researchers simply had to wait to see who got dementia. By the end of the study, 162 women had succumbed. It was then time to look at their drinking habits

The results stood out a mile, showing a "robust protective association" among wine drinkers – as much as a 70% reduction in risk for those who drank wine only, but no effect if they also consumed other alcohols. In fact, the women who predominantly drank beer and spirits had a slightly increased dementia risk. An added bonus for the wine drinkers was that they lived longer.[151]

How much wine did the trick? The Swedes don't give a figure, only reporting that the women's daily intake was "moderate" - hardly surprising given the price of wine in Sweden!

Danish researchers have attempted to find that figure, however. In a study of about 1600 over-65s, drinking up to about 20 grams a day (a quarter of a bottle of wine) was discovered to roughly halve their risk of dementia.[152]

Predictably, the French have also investigated their national drink, which custom demands should accompany main meals. So it's no surprise that this habit persists into old age, with the result that French OAPs often get through a good two-thirds of a bot a day. Far from tut-tutting, as the British medical authorities might well do, French scientists doubtless encourage their old folks with a: "Bravo, allez-y mes vieux!" That's because research by INSERM, the French government research institute, has shown that geriatrics who drink between a quarter and half a litre of wine a day reduce their risk of dementia by a whopping 80%.[153] Incidentally, half a litre of wine a day, although considered OTT in Britain, is deemed "moderate" in France, as the author of the dementia study, Professor Luc Letenneur makes clear in his conclusion that wine must be the key factor in preventing dementia.

> The inverse relationship between moderate wine drinking and incident dementia (is) explained neither by known predictors of dementia nor by medical, psychological or socio-familial factors.

But how to explain these findings?

In 2005, barely noticed by the academic or popular press, Mt. Sinai Medical School in New York played host to one of this century's most bizarre animal experiments. A case of California's best Cabernet Sauvignons was sent direct from Fresno to Manhattan, and served to caged mice. This was not some kind of Animal Rights stunt designed to brighten the laboratory animals' dismal lives, but a serious scientific experiment by expert neuroscientists. What these medical maitre d's wanted to discover was this: can red wine or plain alcohol improve brain function sufficiently to prevent dementia?

In addition to their normal feed, three groups of mice were given either water, water plus pure alcohol, or water plus wine – all allowed to be consumed ad lib. After 7 months, their 'spatial memory' (loosely, intelligence) was tested. The first two groups "performed poorly" but the wine-drinking rats came out way on top.

The fun didn't last, however, as the animals were "sacrificed" so their brains could be examined to see what physical changes the wine had produced. The results were dramatic:

> We found that Cabernet Sauvignon treatments…reduced amyloidogenic Aβ1–40 and Aβ1–42 peptides in the neocortex and hippocampus…(The treatments) also decreased the neocortical Alzheimer's Disease-type amyloid plaque burden.[154]

In plain language, wine had beneficial effects on the brain, in particular by reducing the number of peptides and plaques known to be associated with Alzheimer's Disease (AD).

But humans can also have their brains examined – completely painlessly – via the marvel of MRI brain scans. Once again, completely in line with laboratory animal research, science has discovered that human wine drinkers' brains tend to be healthier than non-drinkers'.

In 2014, for example, Columbia University NY researchers scanned the brains of nearly 600 Northern Manhattan residents over age 65 - some wine drinkers, some teetotallers - with astonishing results:

> Participants who consumed a light-to-moderate amount of total alcohol had larger relative brain volumes than non-drinkers, and this association was likely to be driven by wine consumption. These findings suggest that light to moderate alcohol consumption, in particular wine, is potentially beneficial for brain aging.[155]

But how do these findings translate into the real world? How much wine is needed to ward off dementia? The Danes say a quarter of a bottle a day, and the French say up to two-thirds.

Not to be left behind, the Italians have also weighed in on the question. They have descended on old people's homes, ferreting out both boozers and non-boozers. They rounded up nearly 16,000 seniors and subjected them to "cognitive performance" tests. The findings were pretty bad news for those who didn't drink, almost a third of whom were found to be mentally challenged. "Cognitive impairment was detected in 29% of non-drinkers", the researchers reported, whereas 10% fewer drinkers were affected. How much did the Italians need to drink in order to keep their marbles?

> A daily alcohol consumption of less than 40 g for women and less than 80 g for men.[156]

say the researchers, meaning that up to half a bottle (women) and a full bottle of wine (men) per day maintained mental functioning. The Italian medics add a caveat, however: drink much above those levels and the cognitive benefits tail off.

However, the Brits have put a bit of a dampener on all this. A recent study of over 300,000 Britons showed that the ideal wine intake to prevent dementia is a third of a bottle a day - but only in men, not women.[157]

As these are yet more clear-cut examples of differences between the sexes, perhaps it's about time I explained why men and women differ so markedly in their response to drink.

Summary

Moderate amounts of wine can help prevent dementia - up to a bottle of wine a day for men, and half that for women.

6

Sexism and Racism

Although it may disturb some *bien pensants* to hear it, men and women differ markedly in their response to alcohol. For some reason known only to Mother Nature herself, women are less able to process the same volume of alcohol as men. It follows that, for the same alcohol intake, women will get drunker quicker, and have higher blood alcohol levels than men. Acetaldehyde, the potentially carcinogenic breakdown product of alcohol, may also take longer to be eliminated in women.[158]

The evidence is very consistent: men can safely drink about twice as much alcohol as women, and benefit from it at roughly twice the intake.

That's a huge difference. There are no other autonomic bodily functions that are so different between the sexes - not energy needs, not oxygen requirements, not digestion...nothing.

Why is alcohol so special?

One reason often cited is that women are generally smaller than men and so have less body mass to absorb the alcohol in. That explanation is OK as far as it goes, but women are only slightly smaller than men, not half their size. So that can't be the explanation. The theory has two variants, though: one says that women's bodies contain less water than men's, thus making it more difficult for them to dilute alcohol; the other says that because alcohol is not fat-soluble, and women's bodies contain more fat, *ergo* more alcohol ends up in female blood than men's.

But those arguments don't really wash either, because the amounts of body fat and water aren't that vastly different between the sexes.

There's got to be a more fundamental reason…and there is, but you're going to have to stomach a bit of science.

As soon as you down a drink, your body immediately begins a detoxification process, using two sets of enzymes, which can process about 10 grams of alcohol per hour.

They have complicated scientific names, of course: alcohol dehydrogenase (ADH) and aldehyde dehydrogenase (ADLH).

It's these enzymes that appear to be responsible for the sex differences.

The ADH enzymes are in charge of what's called "first-pass alcohol metabolism", where about 20% of alcohol is broken down in the stomach. Here, there are fairly clear differences between the sexes, with women coming off worst, for the simple reason that they possess fewer of them – particularly women under the age of 40.[159]

But 80% of alcohol processing happens in the liver, where the ALDH enzymes kick in. While alcohol is whizzing around the body in the bloodstream, it's these enzymes that break down alcohol into acetaldehyde and then quickly transform it into harmless acetic acid. Sadly for women, they have far fewer of these enzymes too.[160]

So, science says that women's inability to handle alcohol as efficiently as men is mainly due to having been dealt such a poor hand of alcohol-detoxifying enzymes. If you then add in the sex differences in body weight, water and fat, that ensemble could easily explain why women are so heavily on the boozing losing side.

Nobody has a clue why Mother Nature has so disfavoured her female progeny.

But alcohol isn't only sexist, it's racist too.

Race

Again at the risk of contravening the fashionable tenets of racial equality, I must report that different races also lack these key ADH/ADLH enzymes. Top of the list are Mongoloids (Japanese, Chinese and South-East Asians)[161] [162]; next, native Australians, native Americans and African-Americans [163], distantly followed by Semites.[164] About 50% of Asians and 20% of Semites are affected.

The most obvious effect of these populations' lack of alcohol-detoxifying enzymes is a visual one: their faces flush a deep red when they drink even "the amounts of alcohol that have no detectable effects on Europeans".[165] The flushing is believed to be caused by acetaldehyde, the alcohol metabolite created during the body's alcohol detoxification process. In Europeans, ADH/ADLH enzymes rapidly convert acetaldehyde to harmless acetic acid, but this fairy godmother's magic wand is genetically denied to these populations, seriously delaying the detoxification process.[166]

As it's a mild poison, acetaldehyde makes one feel pretty ropey, so it's no surprise that many of these groups tend to shun alcohol.

Why Europeans are exempt is discussed in my previous book *The Good News About Booze*. Briefly, a possible explanation relates to urbanisation, and cities' potentially contaminated water supplies. In both Greco-Roman and medieval eras, wine and beer respectively were added to drinking water - a happy serendipitous ploy, as our ancestors would have had no scientific knowledge that alcohol kills bacteria and viruses. This would have resulted in selection pressures favouring the survival of people with the most powerful detoxifying enzymes.

Summary

European males are particularly favoured drinkers, as they have powerful alcohol-detoxifying enzymes which, to a greater or lesser extent, women and certain non-European races tend to lack.

7

Weight

This chapter is sure to surprise you. Although wine, like all types of alcohol, 'contains' a lot of calories, the scientific evidence is that it does not put on weight. Strange but true.

Indeed, it was the narrow issue of alcohol and calories that propelled me into the whole question of alcohol and general health. Before that, I had had no real interest in the subject at all, but when I chanced upon the discovery that the health warnings about alcohol causing overweight were wrong, I felt compelled to investigate the science behind the whole subject of the demon drink's effect on health in general.

In this chapter, I'll share my journey of exploration into the paradox of why alcohol, which in theory ought to put on weight, actually doesn't.

The issue

One fact that's been drummed into us is that alcohol is high in calories - almost as high as fat - and is therefore fattening. It's a message harped on by the medical profession who, having scared us with their promulgations about alcohol and health, like to add the *coup de grace* by appealing to our vanity. To fight the flab, they say, ditch the drink (my tag line, not theirs).

Here's what the US Dietary Guidelines tell us:

> Alcohol contributes 7 calories per gram, and...alcohol is a top calorie contributor in the diets of many American adults.[167]

And here's Samara Nielsen, a "nutritional epidemiologist" at CDC's Center for Health Statistics:

> A lot of people don't think about the calories in alcoholic
> beverages. A 12-ounce can of beer is 150 calories, about the
> same as a 12-ounce can of regular soda.[168]

A final blast from the British Nutrition Foundation:

> Most people would baulk at consuming a full glass of single
> cream, but wouldn't think twice about a couple of pints of beer.
> But the calorie content is similar and, over time, excess alcohol
> intake is likely to lead to weight gain.[169]

What's really odd about these statements from some of the
world's top nutritionists is that they contradict the evidence
gathered from the most important, but lowliest 'members' of
their own profession – animals. Most of what nutritionists
claim to know about feeding human beings is derived from
experiments on laboratory rats and mice. For example, literally
thousands of rodents have paid with their lives to establish the
connection between transfats and heart disease.

What about the connection between alcohol and weight?
Well, many fewer animals have been recruited to test that
question – largely I suspect because everyone knew what the
answer would be. After all, alcohol 'contains' lots of calories,
ergo if animals can be persuaded to have a bit of a booze-up,
they will – indeed must - put on weight. What's the point of
confirming the obvious?

Well, in 2008 nutritionists at the prestigious University of
Texas at Austin did want to confirm the obvious. Concerned
by the obesity epidemic among American women, and
believing that alcohol might be a major cause, they wanted to
quantify the problem. So they got hold of a bunch of identical
female mice and split them into two groups: one group's cages
were supplied with ordinary water, while the water in the
others' cages was laced with a hefty dose of 20% alcohol. 20
weeks later, the animals' weights were measured. To the
researchers' utter amazement, although the alcohol-drinking
mice had consumed more 'calories' via the alcohol, they put
on no extra weight at all. "Chronic alcohol consumption did

not increase susceptibility to gaining weight or becoming obese", they reported.[170]

Other researchers have found the same thing. In similar trials on rats, Brazilian nutritionists reported finding that "well-nourished rats cannot utilize alcohol-derived calories."[171] A third example: in a highly controlled year-long experiment, Florida pharmacologists found that alcohol-drinking mice *lost weight* compared to water-drinking mice, even though their calorie intakes were identical.[172]

Some laboratory animals have been lucky enough to be given wine. In 2008 Portuguese biochemists did an experiment testing water, spirits and wine (Douro), administered to three groups of young growing rats. After eight weeks, the water rats had put on 15% more weight than the other two groups, despite similar calorie intakes. Although wine and alcohol were neck and neck in the weight stakes, wine was found to have an important advantage. Examining the animals post-mortem, the researchers made an astonishing discovery: the fat cells in the wine-drinking rats had actually shrunk. The researchers were cock-a-hoop, saying that those results were of "the utmost significance".[173]

Why? Because it's well known that the bigger your fat cells the greater your risk of being overweight.

But would these animal discoveries also apply to humans?

One of the simplest studies was a clinical trial by sports scientists at Colorado State University, who asked this common-sense question: does drinking a couple of glasses of wine a day put on weight or not? A group of men were studied for 12 weeks, during which they either drank a third of a bottle of "13% ABV" (i.e. fairly strong) red wine a day for 6 weeks and then abstained for the next 6 weeks, or vice-versa. The results were crystal-clear:

> In free-living subjects over a 6-week period, the addition of two glasses of red wine to the evening meal does not appear to influence any measured variable which may adversely affect body weight or promote the development of obesity.[174]

But what about wine-drinkers in the real world?

Australia has some fine vineyards, so it's a happy hunting ground for wine research scientists. In a project called the Melbourne Collaborative Cohort Study, the lives of nearly 6000 Aussies were studied to discover how to prevent 'middle-aged spread' - or in researcher-speak: "Predictors of Increased Body Weight and Waist Circumference for Middle-Aged Adults". After a monitoring period of nearly 12 years, the best ways found to keep off the pounds were utterly predictable: "exercise and healthy eating". But less obvious and just as effective was "low to moderate alcohol consumption" - a breakdown of the figures favouring wine in particular.[175]

Even more dramatic findings came in 2012 from another group of people seriously at risk of middle-aged spread – post-menopausal women. In this American study, 15,000 drinkers and non-drinkers (average age 62) were followed for 7 years, and their weights correlated with their alcohol intakes. There were two astonishing findings: first, most weight was gained by the teetotallers, and second, among the drinkers, those who put on the least weight were the heaviest drinkers. Once again, wine was more effective than beer or spirits, with wine drinkers hardly putting on any weight at all. Don't believe me? Here are the relevant quotes from the study:

> Women with the highest intake of alcohol demonstrated the least weight gain over time... Wine consumption showed the greatest protective association for the risk of overweight.[176]

How much wine did these women have to drink to halt middle-aged spread in its tracks? At least 13.5 grams of alcohol a day (a large glass of wine).

However, there's a big caveat here. Not all human studies on wine and weight are quite so clear-cut, with some showing less benefit or indeed no benefit at all. How come? The reason is simple: in population studies it's difficult to disentangle drinking habits from eating habits - not least because drinking can (in old-fashioned pot-smoking jargon) give you 'the munchies'.

The only way round that is to narrow the issue right down, by doing calorie-controlled human clinical trials.

No such trial has been done using wine, but here are the striking results from one done on spirits:

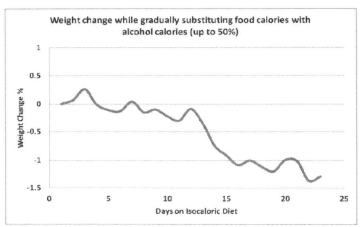

Derived from: Lieber C.S. (1991). Perspectives: do alcohol calories count? *American Journal of Clinical Nutrition,* 54(6), 976-82

This is a graph from a study done way back in 1991. It shows what happened to the average weight of 12 "human subjects" confined for over three weeks under "metabolic-ward conditions". For the first few days, the subjects were given a standard hospital-type diet. On the seventh day, however, food items of a known calorific value were removed from the diet, and substituted by alcohol of exactly the same calorific value. On each subsequent day, more food was removed and substituted by alcohol – again maintaining the subjects' identical calorie intake. The graph shows weight falling as soon as the first food item was replaced with alcohol. The trial ended after two weeks, by which time the calorie value of the food had been halved, so that the subjects were finally ingesting 50% of their total calories from alcohol.

In theory, because their daily calorie intakes were identical throughout the study, the subjects' weights should have remained exactly the same. But no: the more alcohol was substituted for food, the more weight they lost. As the graph shows, they ended up losing almost 1.5% of their weight – a very high figure considering it occurred in just three weeks. The research team were dumbfounded, reporting:

> Chronic consumption of substantial amounts of alcohol is not associated with the expected effect on body weight. [177]

Head-scratching all round, then.. and a real kick in the teeth to the Calorie Theory of weight gain.

How come?

I won't bore with the details of the various explanations for this so-called "alcohol calorie deficit", but here's a summary of the three front-runners:

1. Low Insulin levels. As we saw in chapter 4, alcohol is very good at reducing insulin levels, and it's now well established that the lower one's insulin levels the less glucose is stored as body fat.

2. The Calorie Theory itself. Are calories really a reliable measure of how much various foods will put on weight? I dealt with this issue at length in my last book *The Good News About Booze*, where I showed that the Calorie Theory is based on the idea that the body is like a furnace, and food is like coal. Indeed, believe it or not, the calorie values of individual foods are even today calculated by putting them in a mini-furnace and burning them – a ludicrous proxy for what actually happens to food in the body.

I'm by no means alone in doubting the Calorie Theory. Over the last 70 years, scores of scientists, researchers and science writers like myself have come to the same conclusion - for example, Dr Herman Taller in 1961[178], Professor of Nutrition Jennie Brand-Miller in 2002[179], science writer Gary Taubes in 2008[180], nutrition researcher Dr Zoe Harcombe in 2011[181] and London University Professor Tim Spector in 2020.[182]

3. The Glycemic Index (GI). This relatively new way of analysing foods is steadily gaining ground as an alternative to the Calorie Theory, as it's far more sophisticated. The Index is based on laboratory studies measuring the amount of glucose produced in people's blood after they've eaten individual foods. Glucose is the key measure, because it is primarily surplus glucose which is stored in fat cells in the body, thus contributing to weight gain.[183] Contrary to common - even medical - belief, it's not fat that makes you fat, it's glucose.

The GI uses a scale of 0 to 100 to indicate the least and most glucose-producing foods. In pole position at 100 is sugar, as it's very readily converted into glucose; at the 50 mark are foods such as pulses, beans and wholemeal bread, while at the near zero level are nuts.

Now nuts are a key example of the chasm between the GI and calorie theories. Nuts are full of fat and so score very highly in the 'calorie index'. On the other hand, they produce very little blood glucose, so they score very low in the Glycemic Index. Which of the two indices is correct? Here's the perfect test: if the calorie theory is right, feeding people nuts must result in weight gain; whereas, if the GI theory is right, it should not.

What does the evidence actually show?

The very latest summary of thirty years of research is clear. It lists a wide variety of studies which consistently show that nuts do not increase weight; these studies include Randomised Controlled Trials, the 'gold standard' of evidence.[184] So we now have our answer. The fact that an intake of supposedly 'high calorie' nuts has no effect on weight fires a torpedo into the already sinking ship of the Calorie Theory.

But what have nuts got to do with alcohol, including wine?

Well, right at the bottom of the Glycemic Index - even below nuts - are to be found gin, whisky, vodka and red wine, which all score a resounding 0. Yes, zero. Why? Because none of those drinks has any effect on blood glucose levels, and so cannot increase weight.

As an aside, the only booze exception is beer. That's because beer contains maltose, which is extremely high on the Glycemic Index - hence, the classic 'beer belly'. But you've never heard of a gin belly or a wine belly, have you?

Finally, in case you are in any doubt that alcohol calories don't count, here's what no less an authority than NIAAA, the United States government's top alcohol body, tells us:

> Although alcohol is an energy source, how the body processes and uses the energy from alcohol is more complex than can be explained by a simple calorie conversion value. For example, alcohol provides an average of 20 percent of the calories in the diet of the upper third of drinking Americans, and we might expect many drinkers who consume such amounts to be obese. Instead, national data indicate that, despite higher caloric intake, drinkers are no more obese than non-drinkers. Also, when alcohol is substituted for carbohydrates, calorie for calorie, subjects tend to lose weight, indicating that they derive less energy from alcohol than from food. The mechanisms accounting for the apparent inefficiency in converting alcohol to energy are complex and incompletely understood.[185]

Summary

Wine contains alcohol which, although high in calories, does not put on weight.

The reasons may be that:
1. wine reduces the size of fat cells
2. alcohol reduces insulin levels
3. the basic theory about calories is wrong.

8

Guts

'The gut' is the common name for the twenty feet of convoluted intestinal tubing linking one's stomach to the outside world. Until recently, its functions were believed to be simple: finish off the messy business of food digestion, extract as many nutrients as possible, and expel the remainder as waste. But here's a surprise: although once thought to be a cesspit of harmful bacteria, the gut is now believed to play a vital role in maintaining a healthy body - and even a healthy mind.

And there's another surprise. That exceptionally messy area of the body could well be responsible for at least some of the exceptionally healthy outcomes of wine drinking.

Thanks to modern genetics, we now know the gut harbours a community of about 5000 different species of tiny organisms – mainly bacteria and fungi. There are up to 100 trillion of them, with an astonishing total weight of about two kilograms. Until recently these were thought to be harmful. But no more. Many of these microbes have been discovered to be vital for our health. They do at least two key jobs: extracting the nutrients from food, and producing hundreds of different chemicals designed to support the immune system.

This newly discovered battalion of gut bacteria is the latest thing in nutritional science, triggering a growing slew of studies into the 'microbiome' - the new buzz word for the semi-permanent microbes inhabiting our gut. Why semi-permanent? Because research shows that we ourselves mainly control what types of bacteria live there, simply by deciding what to put in our mouths. For example, at one extreme, oral antibiotics will kill many gut bacteria (explaining why diarrhea is a frequent result of antibiotic use), while 'probiotics' such as fermented foods and yogurt will feed them. In everyday terms though, what largely control our microbiome are the foods we choose to ingest.

The latest research says that the key to a healthy gut is to maintain as diverse a population of bacteria as possible[186] enabling there to be a balance between harmful and beneficial ones. If this is upset, it can lead to "gut dybiosis", causing inflammation both locally and throughout the body.

Professor Tim Spector, Britain's leading microbiome researcher, cites evidence (some of it his own) showing that microbiome diversity is severely reduced by 'ultra-processed food' – mainly because of the sugar, artificial sweeteners, emulsifiers and preservatives which go into its manufacture.[187]

To date, as many as 25 diseases have been associated with an unhealthy microbiome; these include heart disease, diabetes, obesity, dementia and even some cancers.[188]

Ah ha, interesting...! Alert readers will note that these diseases are the very ones prevented by drinking red wine, as outlined in previous chapters.

Happenstance or could there be a connection? Answer: it's no coincidence.

There's rapidly mounting evidence that wine - red especially - is exceptionally good for microbiome health, say two Spanish research teams.[189] [190]

However, the most convincing research data have come from Professor Spector of Kings College London, a man who has devoted much of his life to studying twins. Over the years he has managed to recruit nearly 1500 twins to test various theories about lifestyle and health, with a particular emphasis on the microbiome. Focussing on twins rather than ordinary bods has big advantages: you can rule out genetic and socioeconomic differences when comparing the effects of different dietary interventions.

In the mid 2010s, Spector asked his battalion of twins to keep track of how much alcohol they drank, breaking it down into the main alcohol types (spirits, beer, wine and cider), and then tested their individual gut bacteria. The results were startling: while beer, cider and spirits had no beneficial effects, "there was a significant increase in gut diversity in daily wine drinkers", says Spector.[191] In other words, wine drinkers had the most healthy gut bacteria.[192]

There are two key points to take from Spector's data: 1. white wine isn't nearly as effective as red, doubtless because it contains less of the valuable grape polyphenols. 2. for maximum gut diversity, you've got to drink red wine every day - implying that the gut needs a constant supply of the precious liquid. A glass or two a day is ideal, says Spector, but even quite small amounts are of value.

For example, one of the health problems associated with being carnivorous is that the very process of digesting red meat inevitably creates oxidizing by-products which can be mildly carcinogenic.[193]

Remarkably, scientists at the Hebrew University in Jerusalem found that when people drink quite modest amounts of red wine along with meat, those toxic by-products are significantly reduced.[194]

Other researchers have delved even further into the microbiome, after the discovery that the gut is closely linked to the brain. How come? Well for one thing, there is a major physical connection between the two areas, via the vagus nerve. Interestingly, the communication isn't one way: the gut sends signals to the brain and vice-versa. This is known as the "gut-brain axis". Furthermore, some gut bacteria produce metabolites which are identical to brain chemicals. The most important of these are serotonin, a major mood-altering chemical, and dopamine, the 'reward' chemical. Surprisingly, both these neurotransmitters are thought to be produced almost entirely within the gut, which helps explain why the gut is increasingly being referred to as "the second brain".

But can altering gut bacteria actually affect mental states? The answer is yes. Over the past decade, a growing body of evidence has suggested that "compositional changes in the gut microbiome are highly correlated with several mental disorders", says a 2020 review of the research evidence.[195]

Nutritionists are now actively speculating that a diversely populated gut may explain wine's value in reducing the risk of Alzheimer's disease, for example.[196] [197]

The new microbiome evidence is a significant breakthrough in our understanding of why red wine is so health-promoting, helping to explain the very positive evidence already outlined in this book. It's now known that heart disease, diabetes, obesity, dementia and even some cancers are linked to an unhealthy microbiome, so it stands to reason that a healthy microbiome may do the reverse. "Drinking a moderate amount of red wine daily .... could be a significant factor in explaining (its) health benefits," says Spector.[198]

Summary

Recent nutritional science has discovered that the bacteria living in our gut have profound effects on our health - both causing and preventing a wide range of diseases. Maximum disease prevention occurs when the gut bacteria are maximally diverse. One way to achieve this is by consuming red wine daily.

9

Other Health Benefits

Sexual Function

A few centuries ago, wine and eroticism were fashionable subjects for pictorial art. These paintings usually feature a wine-sodden Bacchus cavorting with flirtatious nude females in sunny sylvan glades. Such depictions may cause the modern male to raise an eyebrow, however, because he has been told that drinking causes 'brewer's droop'* - otherwise known as erectile dysfunction (ED) in medspeak.

But this turns out to be largely bollocks, if you will permit the expression in this context.

Contrary to expectation, genitalia experts have discovered that drinking increases not only desire but also performance. A report by a Taiwanese urologist (with the wonderfully appropriate name of Dr Jiann Bang-Ping) cites a dozen international studies (including his own) demonstrating that male drinkers - of all types of alcohol - have up to half the risk of ED compared to non-drinkers.[199]

As for the female equivalent of ED, wine itself has been shown to be of more value than any other alcohols. The world expert in this relatively unprobed area is Italian researcher Professor Nicola Mondaini. She has conducted surveys on nearly 1000 women in Tuscany, and found that a couple of glasses a day have measurable effects. "Regular moderate intake of red wine is associated with higher...sexual desire, lubrication, and overall sexual function compared to teetotallers", she tells us frankly.[200]

---

* Brewers droop is a genuine phenomenon. The culprit isn't alcohol but the hops in beer which contain estrogen-mimicking compounds.

The Prostate

Women readers, you may skip this, as you haven't got one.

For men, the prostate is a ridiculously annoying organ for the job it has to do - which is simply to add some carrier fluid to sperm during orgasm.

Why annoying? Because the prostate can become troublesome during the everyday activity of peeing, as for reasons known only to the entity that invented it, it may interfere with urine flow. As men get older, the prostate can enlarge and constrict the urinary tract, causing an unwarranted desire to pee…far too often for the victim to lead a peaceful life. This enlargement is called Benign Prostatic Hypertrophy (BPH), although its treatments are far from benign. Surgeons have developed techniques - some more or less invasive and/or painful - to rectify the problem. Sadly, surgical side effects can also include ED.

For less severe cases, there are pharmaceutical drugs to alleviate BPH, but they're not very effective and also have side effects - again including ED.

Happily, wine can come to the rescue.

Once again, it's the Italians who have led the charge. One hospital-based study showed that drinkers had a significantly reduced risk of BPH, and that the risk reduced the more alcohol they imbibed.[201]

Although the researchers didn't mention wine *per se,* you can bet your bottom euro that, because Italian men are primarily wine drinkers, it was wine that did the trick.

A later survey of the international evidence confirmed the good news, finding that all types of alcohol could reduce BPH risk by a substantial 35%, achieved by a minimum alcohol intake roughly equal to a third of a bottle of wine a day.[202]

The other problem with the prostate is cancer, men's major killer after heart disease. But, as shown in chapter 2, wine has no effect on prostate cancer risk one way or the other.

Multiple sclerosis

Wine can also relieve the symptoms of this hideous auto-immune neurological disease. One can only pity the victims (who tend to be female), as the mind is not affected, so they are fully conscious of the gradual disintegration of their bodies…finally ending in death.

Pharmaceutical drugs are pretty ineffective, and in any case come with a raft of side-effects.

In 2016 Harvard doctors decided to test their hunch that alcohol might be valuable, as well as having more pleasant side-effects. They monitored almost a thousand MS patients for a whole year, noting their alcohol intake and MS symptoms. Lo and behold, the drinkers among the patients were found to have almost half the symptoms of the teetotallers. Red wine was found to be particularly effective, with a mere half a glass a day providing rapid symptom relief.

> Our findings add to the increasing amount of literature describing an inverse association between moderate alcohol intake and neurological disability in MS patients, and show similar effects with red wine consumption.[203]

say Harvard.

Arthritis

Another crippling auto-immune disease, for which the pharmaceutical industry can only offer palliation. It won't surprise you to learn that wine can do just as well.

A study on 2000 "severe arthritis" sufferers in Nottingham UK, showed strong evidence that a mere glass of wine a day halved arthritis symptoms, with higher intakes reducing the pain still further. Wine's benefits were objectively confirmed by X-ray.[204]

But, as usual in biological research, not all findings agree. In fact, the vast majority of studies don't show that wine has any special place in arthritis, as all kinds of alcohol will reduce symptoms. The latest summary of the entire research base confirms that drinkers of any alcohol have "significantly lower disease activity" than non-drinkers - a staggering 67% reduction, even among heavy drinkers.[205]

Common Cold

The British government once thought that getting a cold was important enough to warrant setting up a special centre to study it. In the 1980s, the Common Cold Research Unit organised a human trial to test the health effects of tobacco and alcohol, firmly believing that both sinful substances would exacerbate cold symptoms. So the researchers deliberately infected a group of nearly 400 people with five cold viruses (including a corona virus - the one that would be later manipulated to cause the Covid-19 scare), and sat back to watch who succumbed.

To their immense surprise, they found that the drinkers in the group had far fewer cold symptoms than everybody else. Predictably, smokers fared the worst, but so did non-drinkers too, getting as many colds as smokers.[206]

By the way, shortly after this bombshell discovery, the Unit was closed down - coincidence, or punishment for coming up with unacceptable findings?

What about colds and wine drinkers, though? The British study wasn't sophisticated enough to look at wine drinking specifically (probably because Brits didn't drink much wine in the 1980s), but Spanish researchers have since stepped in to fill in the gap.

In a year-long study on nearly 5000 Spaniards, wine drinkers were found to have almost half the risk of catching a cold as teetotallers (yes, despite their fine wines, some Spaniards don't drink them!). In contrast to the British study, however, wine-drinking smokers fared just as well as non-smokers. Once again, non-drinkers were the worst off.[207]

Osteoporosis

Wine is also jolly good news for bones, especially if the bones are fairly old and female, say US researchers. About 2,500 men and women taking part in the long-term Framingham survey group were studied for their drinking habits, and although beer and spirits didn't show much effect on men, older women who drank wine or spirits toughened up important bits of their skeleton:

> Compared to non-drinkers, hip and spine bone mineral densities were significantly greater in postmenopausal women consuming more than 28 grams a day of total alcohol or wine .[208]

Similarly in Romania, an observational study on about 500 people found that anyone - men or women - who drank "moderate" or even "chronic" amounts of wine had half the bone fractures of non-drinkers.[209]

Gallstones

These are nasty balls of stuff (mainly made of cholesterol) which form in the gallbladder, and can block it if they are too numerous. Symptoms can be extreme. A female friend says the pain of a blocked gallbladder is as intense as giving birth.

Once again, wine can come to the rescue…and yet again Italians have paved the way. In the 1980s doctors descended on Castellana, a small town in the heel of Italy, and spent a few years monitoring its 2,000 inhabitants for signs of developing gallstones. Sure enough, wine drinkers were found to have a significantly reduced risk of the disease compared to non-drinkers.[210]

Since then, over twenty further studies have been conducted across the world, collectively showing that drinkers in general have a roughly 40% reduced risk of gallstones, with 40 - 50 grams of alcohol (= two-thirds of a bottle of wine) being the most beneficial daily intake. But higher intakes are almost as effective.[211]

Kidney Stones

Another type of stone, which can develop in the kidneys. It's not totally clear why this occurs, but it's probably due to a kidney malfunction causing a painful build-up of little balls of calcite or uric acid. Although once relatively rare, this disease is rapidly increasing in step with rising levels of obesity. Over 12% of Americans will succumb to it at some stage in their lives.

Once again, Harvard University has been able to draw on the findings from their massive 'lifestyle and health' survey of health professionals. Over a four-year period in the late 1980s, researchers kept tabs on the incidence of kidney stones among the 80,000 women in the survey group. Roughly 1% of them contracted the disease - so 99% didn't. It was then the job of the researchers to see what aspects of their lives prevented the majority from succumbing.

Way top of the list of preventive behaviours was drinking wine, distantly followed by tea and coffee. By the way, grapefruit juice was a no-no, substantially increasing risk. How much wine? Well, although the researchers don't actually specify it, their figures show the more wine the merrier.[212]

Eyes: Macular Degeneration

This progressive disease of the retina often afflicts people as they get older, and can even result in blindness. No-one knows why MD occurs nor how to prevent it. Towards the end of the last century, University of Washington DC ophthalmologists decided to cast a beady eye over the drinking habits of their patients, fully expecting to find that the demon drink would be a major risk factor, but "surprisingly" found the opposite, reporting that:

> Moderate wine consumption is associated with decreased odds of developing age-related macular degeneration. This is an important addition to the current scientific knowledge about MD.[213]

Eyes: Cataracts

This clouding of the pupil is an almost inevitable part of ageing, hitting most people eventually. But its onset can be delayed by wine. A five year study in Iceland found that wine drinkers had half teetotallers' risk of succumbing.[214]

A couple of much bigger, longer-term studies in the UK weren't quite so dramatic, but also confirmed wine's benefits, reporting:

> Compared with non-drinkers, the risk of [needing] incident cataract surgery was [up to] 23% lower among those in the highest category of red wine consumption.[215]

Teeth and Gums

Red wine also has unexpected benefits in the mouth, where it combats plaque[216] - the whitish sticky stuff that tends to coat unbrushed teeth and gums. Plaque is the primary cause of both caries (holes in the tooth enamel) and gum disease, so swilling your mouth out with red wine before downing it could avoid trips to the dentist.

It would be interesting to examine the mouths of professional wine tasters, who only rinse their mouth with wine and never swallow - to avoid getting tiddly. Might another secret reason be to improve oral health?

Summary

Alcohol in general and wine in particular can provide a wide variety of individual health benefits.

10

Living Longer

The last few chapters have shown that wine drinking can reduce your risk of cancer, heart disease, diabetes, obesity and dementia. So it won't surprise you to learn that wine also helps you live longer.

The first person to discover that drinkers in general have longer life expectancies than teetotallers was the celebrated British epidemiologist, Sir Richard Doll, the man who unearthed the link between smoking and lung cancer in the 1960s. It was his pioneering work which kick-started all the public health campaigns about the dangers of tobacco. After tobacco, Doll then turned his attention to alcohol, doubtless expecting to find similar adverse health consequences. However, he found none. In fact to his surprise, he discovered an "inverse effect" on health – that drinkers have a reduced risk of heart disease in particular. He also found that drinkers outlive non-drinkers by a large margin.[217]

However, in marked contrast to his tobacco research, Doll's two key discoveries about alcohol's health benefits were neither publicised nor acted upon.

What a surprise.

The first group to look at longevity in wine drinkers in particular came from Denmark. In a 1995 study published in the British Medical Journal, scientists at the University of Copenhagen reported findings so astonishing that I must quote directly from the journal:

Subjects: 6051 men and 7234 women aged 30-70 years.

Main outcome measure: Number and time of cause-specific deaths from 1976 to 1988.

Results: The risk of dying steadily decreased with an increasing intake of wine - from a relative risk of 1.00 for the subjects who never drank wine to 0. 51 (95% confidence interval 0-32 to 0.81) for those who drank three to five glasses a day.[218]

In plain English, wine drinkers' mortality risk was roughly half that of teetotallers.

Five years later, the Danes repeated the study on a much larger group of people (nearly 25,000), whose mortality rates had been followed for 20 years.[219]

Here's what they found in graph form:

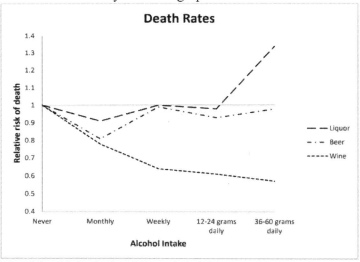

Adapted from M. Grønbaek et al. Type of Alcohol Consumed and Mortality from All Causes, Coronary Heart Disease, and Cancer, *Annals of Internal Medicine*, September 19, 2000 vol. 133 pp 6 411-419

The mortality rates of non-drinkers is the centre line, against which are plotted the death rates of the three types of drinkers.

The differences are stark. For liquor/spirits there is a very slight decrease in mortality at very low intakes, but at higher intakes (about 5 shots of gin/whisky/vodka a day) the mortality risk climbs by 40%. Beer fares much better, but at modestly high intakes (about 3 pints of beer a day) the mortality benefit tails off. Wine, however, stands out as having a massive longevity benefit – and an increasing one, reducing mortality risk by about 40% at intakes of up to roughly a bottle of wine a day.

That steadily plunging death rate seems to imply 'the more the merrier' in terms of wine-drinkers' longevity, but common-sense says there must be a point at which wine's health benefit goes into reverse. So, what's the ideal wine intake for maximum lifespan?

Start intoning "O sole mio", for the answer comes from La Bella Italia.

Italy is one of the world's top wine-drinking nations (possibly because its wines are so good), and its medical statisticians are among the world's leading experts in alcohol research. Put the two together and you get some fascinating research findings.

One example was published in 1995, reporting the results of a huge survey which asked a very simple question: are drinkers healthier than non-drinkers? To the American or British medical authorities, the answer would have been a foregone conclusion. Clearly, drinking no alcohol at all is bound to be healthier than indulging in the demon drink.

But that's not what the Italian scientists discovered - in fact, they found precisely the reverse. Drinkers were much healthier than non-drinkers.

In case you think I'm making this up, I'm once again going to hit you with the summary text of their findings word for word, with two tiny irrelevant bits removed:

> We used data from...58,462 adults aged 25 years and over who are representative of the general Italian population, to compare the prevalence of 16 major chronic diseases or groups of diseases in alcohol abstainers and...current drinkers. We found elevated odds ratios among alcohol abstainers for diabetes, hypertension, myocardial infarction, other heart diseases,

anaemias, gastroduodenal ulcer, cholelithiasis, liver cirrhosis, urolithiasis, and renal insufficiency.[220]

In plain English: compared to alcohol-drinking Italians, we found that non-drinkers have more diabetes, high blood pressure, heart attacks and general heart problems, anemia, stomach ulcers, gallstones, cirrhosis of the liver (*sic!*), urinary tract stones and kidney problems.

Astonishing.

Just as astonishing were the results of another Italian study, one specifically on longevity.

The "male inhabitants" of two villages in Northern and Central Italy were chosen as the medical database, and for thirty long years the men were kept tabs on, with their lifestyles recorded in some detail. By the end of the study, two-thirds of them had died, giving the researchers ample data to compare lifestyles and lifespan. What did they find?

Unsurprisingly, one of the chief causes of premature death was tobacco. But having got that out of the way (in sciencespeak, "after adjusting for smoking"), the men's longevity was found to depend on two main factors: 1. their occupation, and 2. their wine intake.

So who lived longest?

In pole position were those with physically demanding jobs (builders, farmworkers etc.), who also drank about half a bottle of wine a day. Interestingly, however, the less strenuous the job, the more wine was needed to maximize lifespan. In second place were men whose jobs involved "light physical activity" (shop/office workers etc.), but again they had to have drunk "85 to 120 grams of alcohol" (i.e. between a bottle and a litre of wine) a day. The longevity benefit was substantial, giving these men almost six extra years of life compared to people who rarely drank. The researchers acknowledge that downing a litre of wine a day might seem "excessive" in other countries, but emphasise that it was "consumed mostly during meals, following a typical Italian pattern".[221]

However, before you're tempted to raise too many glasses to the Italians, you should be aware that other studies disagree, finding wine's longevity benefits tend to decline at those high Italian intakes. Nevertheless, they all confirm wine's special status as a lifespan booster [222], with consistent findings in France [223] [224] and the USA.

For example, in 2003 a team led by Dr. Arthur Klatsky at Oakland's Kaiser Permanente Medical Center in California reported the results of a 20-year study on 128,000 people, designed to measure the effects of wine intake on overall health and subsequent mortality. Again, I'm driven to give you his verbatim conclusions, as they are so unequivocal:

> The major finding in these data was the independent relation of wine drinking frequency to lower total mortality risk. Perhaps most convincing was the lower risk associated with wine drinking frequency at each of three total drinking levels: less than one glass, one or two glasses, and three or more glasses per day. The reduction in wine-related risk was clearest for deaths attributed to coronary disease and respiratory causes. The unexpected strength and consistency in our data raises the likelihood of a causal association. [225]

In other words, says that last line, we've pretty well proved that wine helps you live longer.

The Californian data closely match what Italian researchers say is the ideal wine intake for optimal health and longevity. First and foremost, they have shown that wine is a key component of the Mediterranean Diet, which itself is now widely acknowledged as the world's healthiest dietary regime. [226]

In fact, say the Italians, standing atop the Med Diet's ingredients (olive oil, fish, unrefined cereals, fruit, vegetables etc.), in prime position is "moderate" wine drinking, representing almost 15% of the Med Diet's health benefits. What's their definition of "moderate"? Up to almost a bottle of wine a day for men, and half that for women. [227]

Seniors' quality of life

"What a drag it is getting old", says the Rolling Stones lyric. One of the biggest drags is losing the ability to do simple tasks – 'functional impairment' in medspeak. Wine can help here too, say Spanish researchers, who have found it can reduce impairment by up to 70%. The key is a "Mediterranean drinking pattern, defined as moderate alcohol intake, with wine preference and drinking only with meals." The evidence is strongest for men drinking about half a bottle of wine a day, and a third of a bottle for women, but larger intakes are almost as convincingly beneficial.[228]

Older but sicker?

Some critics of the longevity evidence have asked: what's the point of living longer if you're ill all the time?...the implication being that a lifetime of drinking – even in moderation – must ultimately catch up with you.

The official medical term for having a healthy old age is the rather poetic "successful ageing", and it's an issue alcohol researchers have been keen to investigate. After all, if daily moderate drinking simply prolongs lives at the expense of underlying health, no-one's going to benefit – neither drinkers themselves nor the wider society in picking up the extra health-care bills.

What's the actual evidence? Well, there's not much information on wine drinking and successful ageing, but there is quite a lot of evidence about alcohol in general.

Harvard University has been best placed to study drinkers' long-term health because many years ago it had the foresight to persuade thousands of 'health professionals' to allow their health records and lifestyle behaviours to be monitored for almost their entire lives. Harvard's famous Nurses Health Study on (ultimately) over 110,000 women was begun in 1976, and by 2012, 13,894 of them had reached the age of 70. Some had been drinkers all their lives, others lifetime abstainers. The researchers wanted to see which group of 70 year-olds was experiencing successful ageing, defined as "being free of eleven major chronic diseases and having no major cognitive impairment, physical impairment, or mental health limitations".

The findings were extraordinary. Health-wise, the worst off were the teetotallers. Compared to their zero alcohol intake,

> Alcohol consumption was associated with a 24% increased odds of successful ageing [at an intake of] 30 to 45 grams of alcohol a day, and 28% at 15 to 30 grams a day.[229]

Harvard found it was the regular drinkers who came off best:

> Independent of total alcohol intake, participants who drank alcohol at regular patterns throughout the week had somewhat better odds of successful ageing: 29% better for those drinking 3-4 days per week, and 47% for 5-7 days per week.

So in contrast to officialdom's strictures to lay off the booze for two or three days a week, the scientific evidence says that regular (almost daily) drinking is the best way to maximize alcohol's health benefits in the old.

In 2006, Australian academics concluded a similar exercise on over 14,000 of their own old ladies, and found almost precisely the same:

> Women who did not consume alcohol were 94% more likely to die than women who drank 10 to 20 grams of alcohol per day, 3 to 6 days per week. Or if the non-drinkers survived, they had lower health-related quality-of-life scores.[230]

How much should oldies drink for maximum benefit? Once again, the answer comes from Denmark, where a goodly number of seniors are fairly heavy drinkers. No surprise that might have got Danish medics worried.

They needn't have been.

Research studies on thousands of Danes stretching over two decades have shown that the over 50s have to drink a serious amount - 70 grams of alcohol (the equivalent of a bottle of wine) a day - before their mortality rate equals that of teetotallers.[231]

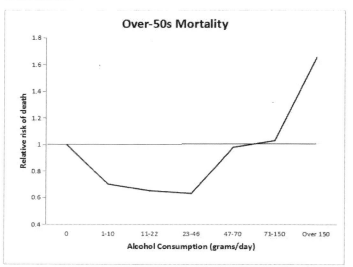

Derived from: Grønbaek M et al (1998) Alcohol and mortality: is there a U-shaped relation in elderly people? *Age and Ageing* ; 27: 739-744

There have been very similar findings in Holland, where a 40 year-long study found that older wine drinkers (in all social classes) outlived non-drinkers by a substantial margin, reporting that:

> Long-term wine consumers had about 5 years longer life expectancy at age 50 compared with no alcohol users.[232]

Interesting stuff, but how does wine do it?

In 2020, an unusual small-scale experiment was done on a group of middle-aged Spanish nuns. They were chosen because they were pretty well teetotallers, not having touched a drop for over two years. So, in more ways than one, they were biologically virgin territory. Every day, they were given a total of half a bottle of red wine with meals - incidentally, described as a "moderate" daily intake. After two weeks, they provided blood and urine samples, which the researchers then analysed for any changes in the women's "longevity-associated genes". The results were stunning:

> The major conclusions of our study are that moderate wine consumption increases the expression of p53, sirtuin1, catalase, and superoxide dismutase - all key longevity-associated genes.[233]

reported the University of Valencia scientists.

UK Biobank

To wrap up this chapter, I want to present you with the latest evidence from the UK Biobank project. This is a unique database of the lifestyle and health records of about half a million Britons, who have all volunteered to allow their lives to be monitored in fairly intimate medical detail. This enormous database has attracted epidemiologists from all over the world to plunder its riches.

The issue is this: since 2016, officialdom has repeatedly claimed that the evidence for alcohol's harms is becoming stronger by the day, warning us that "there is no safe level of drinking", and that any "supposed" health benefits from drinking are "an old wives' tale".[234]

In short, we are exhorted to believe that it would be far better for everyone's health if we all became teetotal or switched to zero alcohol drinks.

But does the latest data from such a robustly evidential source as the Biobank support this?

Here are three scientific reports since 2020, all of which have examined the lifespan of drinkers in the Biobank cohort.

In 2021, after tracking the Biobankers' health for nine whole years, a group of US researchers reported:

> We found that healthy drinking habits - i.e. regular drinking more than 4 days a week and drinking with meals - were associated with lower risks of all-cause mortality and cause-specific mortality ....with lower risks among those consuming more than 50 grams/week and less than 300 grams/week.[235]

Let's unpack those grams/week figures. Rephrased, they show that alcohol's longevity benefits start to kick in at a maiden aunt's daily level of consumption: a very small gin/whisky, ditto glass of wine, or a third of a pint of beer a day. But the benefits continue at more muscular intakes - up to 300 grams of alcohol a week, i.e. 43 grams of alcohol per day. That's two pints of fairly strong beer, three measures of spirits, and more than half a bottle of wine. Those amounts are way in excess of many governments' drinking guidelines, of course. Furthermore, the finding that the healthiest drinking pattern is to quaff on more than four days per week again flies in the face of officialdom's strictures.

That study was on alcohol in general, but others show it's much the same story with wine-drinking itself.

Another 2021 Biobank report by a group of Scottish researchers found that:

> Red wine drinking, consumption with food and spreading alcohol intake over 3–4 days were associated with lower risk of mortality and vascular events among regular alcohol drinkers.[236]

Finally, a 2023 Biobank study conducted by German researchers found that:

> In all participants and in both sexes separately, wine intake was not significantly associated with cancer mortality...Light to moderate consumption of wine...was associated with decreased all-cause and non-cancer mortality.[237]

So the evidence about alcohol in general and wine in particular, far from becoming more worrying as the years have gone by, is robustly continuing to confirm that moderate drinking - at intakes which often contradict official guidance - is exceptionally good for one's health.

Summary

Contrary to the official propaganda, drinking alcohol - and wine in particular - continues to have significant health benefits, as evidenced by drinkers' increased lifespan.

11

What's in Wine?

With all the growing evidence for wine's health benefits, what precisely does wine contain to account for them?

Most of wine's constituents are water and alcohol, of course, but the liquid contains a huge array of natural chemicals derived from grapes. Let me quote an expert from the 1980s, an era when scientists wrote in half-way decent prose:

> Wine is a chemical symphony composed of ethyl alcohol, several other alcohols, sugar, other carbohydrates, polyphenols, aldehydates, ketones and pigments, with half a dozen vitamins, fifteen to twenty minerals, more than twenty-two organic acids, and other things that have not yet been identified.[238]

said Dr. Maynard Amerine, Professor of Oenology and Viticulture at UC Davis (the USA's top wine research centre) back in 1986. But wine science has seriously moved on since then. We now know wine contains the following vitamins and minerals:

Thiamine	Calcium Chloride	Iron
Riboflavin	Silicic Acid	Boron
Niacin	Fluoride	Iodine
Choline	Aluminium	Copper
Magnesium	Manganese	Rubidium
Potassium	Sodium	Betaine

Of course, these micronutrients are in very small amounts, but they're still at useful health levels.

But it's not those constituents that have got modern nutritionists excited, it's these:

Polyphenols in Wine
Milligrams per litre

Compound	Red Wine	White Wine
Nonflavonoids	240-500	160-260
Hydroxybenzoicacids	0-260	0-100
p-Hydroxybenzoicacid	20	_
Gallic acid	116	1.4
Total gallates	40	7
Syningic acid	5	_
Protocatechuric acid	88	_
Hyproxycinnamic acids	162	130-154
cls/trans-Coutaric	20	1.8
cls/trans-Caftaric	25	5
Caffeic acid	8.5	2.8
Coumaric acid	12.6	1.5
Ferulic acid	19	_
Stilbenes	750-1060	25-30
trans-Resveratrol	12.3	1.8
Flavonoids	1.0	0.22
Quercetin	18.8	0
Myricetin	16.1	0
Kamempferol	8	0
Rutin	6.8	0
Flavanols	168	15-30
Catechin	57.3	17.3
Epicatechin	89	13.6

I make no apology for peppering your pages with such recondite chemical names – they at least serve to demonstrate wine's multifarious contents. But why are they so interesting to nutritionists?

Because these natural chemicals within wine are all classified as polyphenols…compounds thought to be rather good news for health.

Polyphenols are substances naturally produced by plants in order to protect themselves from stressors such as disease and the ultraviolet rays in sunshine. By the end of the last century, science had begun to discover that polyphenols are valuable health-promoting 'antioxidants' – not just for plants but humans too.

An explanatory diversion. What's wrong with oxidants that they need antis?

Well, the culprit is believed to be a group of chemicals called free radicals. These sound like wayward political renegades, and in a sense biologically they are, because they're dangerous loose cannons. Free radicals are created naturally as a by-product of us being oxygen-breathing, food-eating animals, and, unless they are neutralized, they will damage healthy cells by robbing them of vital electrons. Free radicals can damage DNA and make LDL cholesterol more likely to clog up arteries; they're even thought to be responsible for some cancers and even the ageing process itself.

So the body's free radicals need clobbering. But how? The principal weapons are antioxidants, which we derive from eating plants. Originally, it was thought that fruits, vegetables and cereals were the only source of antioxidants, but as the evidence has built up about wine's health benefits, nutritionists now think we have a hitherto unsuspected extra supply of antioxidant goodies - the polyphenols in wine.

In fact, it turns out that wine has some of the best antioxidants around.

In 1999, British researchers at Guy's Hospital Medical School in London compared the antioxidant properties of wine against standard fruits and vegetables….with remarkable results. They reported finding that:

> The antioxidant activities of 1 glass (150 ml) of red wine are equivalent to 4 apples, 5 portions of onion, 5.5 portions of eggplant, and 3.5 glasses of blackcurrant juice.[239]

That is an astonishing finding. Alone, it shows that a small glass of red wine will more than fulfil the ubiquitous government-mandated "5-a-day" fruit and vegetable regimes.

By the way, the British medics also found that a glass of white wine didn't come close, with it containing one twelfth of the antioxidants in red. Why? As explained earlier, the principal reason is that red wine is made from the entire grape - juice, skin, seeds, pulp, and even grape stems - whereas white wine is made only from the juice.

Resveratol

Wine polyphenols got everyone excited. From early on, the polyphenol that stood out from the crowd was a compound called resveratrol (RSV) – possibly because red wine contains quite a lot of it, and white wine almost none

The first RSV study was done in 1978. By 2023, the number stood at over 17,000 research papers..

Here's an extract from a 2020 paper summarizing the findings:

> Resveratrol has antioxidant, anti-inflammatory, immunomodulatory, glucose and lipid regulatory, neuroprotective, and cardiovascular protective effects, It can protect against chronic diseases such as cardiovascular disease, cancer, liver disease, obesity, diabetes, Alzheimer's disease, and Parkinson's disease.[240]

However, all this is possibly hype. Yes, RSV has caused these protective effects - principally in laboratory test-tubes, and to a certain extent in mice and rats. But in practice it's not been very effective with human beings. That's mainly because RSV is not very "bioavailable" - in other words it's poorly absorbed by the body. As a result, RSV "has made only marginal progress in cancer therapy", for example.[241]

In any case, all this research on RSV is all very well, but it's pretty well valueless for wine drinkers. Here's why.

Although RSV is a major ingredient of red wine, there's in practice not enough of it in a bottle to deliver any significant health benefits. For example, a clinical trial showing that RSV is "effective in improving glycemic control in diabetes"[242] used a daily dose of 250 milligrams of RSV - the amount in 20 litres of wine. Undrinkable and unthinkable.

Another example: in one study, RSV showed some mild benefit for Alzheimers disease, but the old folk needed to ingest up to 1000 milligrams a day of the stuff.[243]

So, how to explain red wine's health benefits? If they're not due to RSV, what else could be responsible?

I'm now going to introduce you to another potent ingredient of wine which you've almost certainly never have heard of. But I predict that, in the years to come, it may become as familiar to wine buffs as RSV. It's another tongue-twister.

Hydroxytyrosol

Shortened to HT, this is a compound widely found in the plant kingdom, and is rapidly being acknowledged as "one of the strongest dietary antioxidants". [244] In fact, it's becoming increasingly recognised as a major reason for the health-giving properties of the Mediterranean diet, as it's found in both olive oil and wine - its two key components.

HT has already chalked up some some remarkable health benefits. Here's a 2020 summary:

> HT is claimed to exert many bioactive properties, including antioxidant, anti-inflammatory, anti-cancerogenic, neuroprotective, immunomodulatory, cardioprotective, anti-diabetic, cytoprotective, antimicrobial, antiviral, endothelial and vascular regulatory, and skin protective properties. Regarding prevention of cardiovascular diseases, in addition to its antioxidant capacity, HT is also claimed to inhibit platelet aggregation, chronic cardiac toxicity, the expression of proteins related to ageing, as well as attenuation of the metabolic alterations of glucose, triglyceride and total cholesterol.[245]

All that medical lingo boils down to one simple thing: HT is damn good for one's general health. So, what's the best way of getting the stuff down one's throat so it can do all those good things to one's body?

Well, although olive oil contains more HT than wine, in practice your salad would literally need to be drowning in vinaigrette for you to get a clinically meaningful dose. The fact is that no-one drinks olive oil for pleasure, whereas of course wine is the complete reverse.

Red wine is a good source of HT, containing about 5 mg per litre[246] so it's one of wine's most abundant antioxidants. It's also more bioavailable than other polyphenols such as RSV - in fact, up to 100% of HT is absorbed by the body[247]. Furthermore, it becomes an even more powerful antioxidant when combined with alcohol[248], so its presence in wine gives it an extra boost.

That's quite a list of 'firsts' for a relatively novel compound, which is why HT is attracting such attention in academia. I'll return to it later in chapter 13.

However, the hoop-la about HT is somewhat bucking the trend in scientific wine circles.

Beyond RSVand HT

There's a growing realisation that, because wine's health benefits are so robust, they're unlikely to be due to the action of single ingredients. Rather, that wine's constituents should be seen more holistically, with them all behaving synergistically - as a mutually reinforcing family of complex "bioactives".

Here's Professor Ramon Estruch at the University of Barcelona on the subject:

> The beneficial effects of moderate wine consumption may be attributed to the overall mix of all of its components and not to a specification of one, such as resveratrol. Indeed, progress can be achieved in the health effects of polyphenols when the one-dimensional antioxidant view of polyphenols is replaced by a view considering their multifaceted bioactivity, as polyphenols are versatile bioactives rather than mere antioxidants.[249]

Indeed. This is the view of the late Professor Gerald Weissmann of New York University:

When it comes to finding treatments for complex diseases, the answers are sometimes right there waiting to be discovered in unexpected places... like the wine racks of the nearest store. The profound impact that the antioxidants in red wine have on our bodies is more than anyone would have dreamt just 25 years ago. As long as [it is] taken in moderation, all signs show that red wine may be ranked among the most potent 'health foods' we know.[250]

"Polyphenols are medicine; is it time to prescribe red wine for our patients?" ask Professors Alfredo Cordova and Bauer Sumpio, cardiologists at America's prestigious Yale University, answering their own question by recommending their fellow doctors to

encourage regular and moderate consumption of red wine, perhaps one or two drinks a day with meals.[251]

Summary

Wine's special health benefits are due to its polyphenol contents, with red wine containing far more than white. Resveratrol is the best researched polyphenol, but there are doubts about how much the body can in practice make use of. Despite having discovered another potent ingredient in hydroxytyrosol, researchers now think that it's the totality of wine's antioxidant ingredients that may account for its health-promoting qualities.

12

Even Healthier Wine

This book has already revealed startling evidence of the health benefits of drinking wine. But can they be improved upon?

In a word, yes. Not so much to do with the wine itself, but how it's produced. Because the brutal fact is that wine-making requires the use of lots of toxic chemicals, most of them man-made.

First, chemicals are widely used in the vineyards themselves. Those lush vines we admire on sunny hillsides only look healthy because they may have been sprayed as many as 25 times in a growing season. The reason is that, for all its romance, wine-growing is highly intensive agriculture - crudely put, despite the sunny open air, wine grapes are factory-farmed. Furthermore, the charmingly neat rows of vines are quintessential monocultures, and monocultures breed disease and infestation.

Whole vineyards can be blighted by fungal diseases such as mildews and grey mould (botrytis), and attacked by creepy-crawlies like nematodes, caterpillars, mealybugs, leafrollers, flea beetles and berry moth larvae. In the last 100 years, agrochemists have developed increasingly effective chemicals to combat them. But with efficacy has come increased toxicity - to both pests and people. So wine grapes are now among the most pesticide-intensive crops in the world.[252]

The other way chemicals can get into wine is during the fermentation process, when the natural yeasts on the grape skins interact with the sugars in the juice to produce alcohol - and hence wine. So far so natural, but wine-makers can also add up to 60 ingredients - to "prevent spoilage", "add clarity", "reduce acidity" and "add flavour". None of these are man-made chemicals, and are often removed before bottling. So they are not considered to be a health risk…..apart from one family of chemicals: the Sulphites.

The Sulphite Saga

The most common additives in wine, sulphites are used as preservatives both after grape harvest and in the wines themselves. Because of their perceived toxicity, their presence in wine must be legally declared, but only above a certain minimum level (10mg per litre). Hence the almost universal "contains sulphites" warning on labels.

But just how toxic are they?

For the vast majority of drinkers, sulphites appear to have no adverse health consequences, but for some people they can cause quite serious health problems. Such unfortunates are exclusively asthmatics and predominantly female. Sulphites can trigger asthma attacks severe enough to be fatal. That's why in 1986 the US Food and Drug Administration banned their use as preservatives on fresh fruits and vegetables, and mandated a label declaration on wine bottles containing more than ten parts per million - a regulation adopted worldwide.

So, apart from asthmatics, need wine drinkers in general be worried?

The most common accusation levelled against sulphites in wine is that they cause headaches.

However, there is very little research to confirm this, with only one small study on the issue. Conducted in Portugal in 2019, it showed that susceptible people could distinguish between low and high sulphite wines, in terms of which produced the worse headaches.[253]

Nevertheless, most studies claim there's no connection,[254] partly because it's red rather than white wine that tends to cause headaches, and yet reds are generally lower in sulphites than whites and sparkling wines - 160 parts per million, 210 ppm. and 250ppm respectively.

Still, many drinkers believe sulphites to be harmful, which is one factor that has led to the growing popularity of a health revolution in wine-making: organic viticulture.

Organic Wines

As recently as the 1960s, organic agriculture was mocked as 'muck and mystery' farming - a term derived from its use of animal manure as fertiliser, plus a few woo-woo ideas like 'working with nature rather than against it.'

It took a consumer revolt against conventional agriculture, with its high use of nutrient-depleting fertilisers and toxic pesticides, to put a stop to insults about organic farming - often from the mouths of top agronomists. After all, muck and mystery is simply the 'mixed farming' system that had existed for thousands of years before the advent of the agrochemical industry.

Organic produce has now become highly prized by the world's middle-class, who are prepared to pay a premium for fruits and vegetables with more flavour and nutrients, and zero (in theory) pesticide residues.

It wasn't long before the wine trade cottoned onto the commercial opportunities of producing organic wines for their well-heeled, health-savvy clients.

Today, organic wine now accounts for roughly 4% of the world wine market. The leading country is Spain, with about 9% of its vineyards now *biologico,* but France, Italy, and Germany are close behind.

What's behind this mini-revolution? It's partly the European Union, with its highly regulated, 'directive'-driven agricultural policies. It's not that the EU has mandated organic viticulture (yet), but its pesticide regulations (going by the name of Integrated Pest Management) are now in practice so onerous that many vineyards find themselves being pretty well *de facto* organic. So it's an open door for growers to go the whole way to full organics.

Unquestionably, the most striking result of this EU legislation is to put a cap on the use of pesticides, including the world's most controversial agrochemical, glyphosate. In 2015, the WHO classified it as both "genotoxic" and "probably carcinogenic to humans". Widely used to kill weeds and grasses around the base of vines, glyphosate has been claimed not to find its way into the wines themselves, but this is now known to have been a self-serving delusion. In France, growers who decide to go organic are often prevented from doing so because of the residues from past glyphosate sprayings, which not only still remain in the ground, but also end up in their wines[255] ... Lord alone knows how much glyphosate wine drinkers have been unknowingly ingesting over the years.

Not to be outdone, California has also joined the organic revolution - albeit hesitantly, with less than 3% of its vineyards now organic.

Zero pesticides in your glass (in theory) is all very well, but do organic wines taste better than conventional wines? To answer that, a UCLA team studied the wine-tasting records of three leading US wine magazines which had employed top wine masters as their wine tasters. Over a ten year period, a grand total of nearly 75,000 wines from nearly 4000 Californian vineyards had been blind-tasted...with clear-cut results. On average, "wine quality ratings" were 4.1% higher for organic than conventionally produced wines.[256]

But what does that mean for drinkers' health? Well, it's too early - as well as too impractical - to tease out whether organic wine drinkers are any healthier. However, it goes without saying that a guaranteed (again, in theory) pesticide-free drink must be intrinsically better for health.

The other benefit of organic Californian wines is a significantly reduced content of sulphites. State regulations say that organic wines must not exceed 10 parts per million.*

The same doesn't apply to Europe, however, where there are no such strictures: organic wines are allowed to contain ten times that amount.

What about organics in the rest of the world? South Africa and Australia are pretty poor, with less than 2% of vineyards having gone organic, but New Zealand claims a remarkable 10%.

The big laggard is Latin America, with only a handful of vineyards now *biologico*. This is hardly surprising as there is not much push from individual governments to limit pesticide use. Unsurprisingly, South American wines tend to contain the highest amounts of pesticides in the world.[257]

Biodynamics

There's another revolution in healthy viticulture: super-duper organic wine-making. It uses an agricultural system created in the 1920s by (of all people) a religious philosopher - a calling unlikely to fit one for grubby farming.

The philosopher/farmer was an Austrian called Rudolf Steiner. He called himself an "anthroposophist" - Greek for 'the study of man'. However, Steiner's real interests were not so much with man himself, but more with man's relationship with Planet Earth - and indeed the whole Cosmos. The practical expression of this was his invention of a remarkable agricultural system he called biodynamic farming, designed to "unite soil, plant, animal and human health with cosmic and Earthly influences."

Steiner's biodymanics set some bizarre rules. For example, farmers had to time the sowing and harvesting of crops according to lunar and planetary positions. Even odder was the

---

* Some growers get round this regulation by labelling their wines as "made from organically grown grapes" - deliberately saying nothing about the wine's contents.

requirement to make fertiliser out of cow dung (fair enough), but only after the dung had been stuffed into hollow cow horns and buried in the ground for 6 months (wow, where did that come from?). Equally bizarrely, Steiner claimed that the contents of a single cow horn would fertilise a whole acre, if diluted in enough "energised" water.

But don't mock. Surprisingly, the soils on biodynamic farms have been found to be just as fertile as those on 'straight' organic farms, despite the latter using a far greater volume of animal manure-based composts.

During Steiner's lifetime, a few vineyards adopted his quasi-mystical practices, but they all seem to have died out. Currently, the world's oldest biodynamic vineyard is claimed to be in the Sud-Tyrol hills on the Austrian/ Italian border. Founded in the 1970s by Rainer Loacker, it's now run by his two sons Franz and Hayo.

To the outsider, the vineyard looks like any other, except that the rows of vines are planted a bit wider than usual, and there's low-lying vegetation everywhere. Some wine-growers might have been tempted to glyphosate that up, but it's all valuable stuff, Hayo told me. The vegetation is made up of deliberately sown plant species, specifically chosen for their deep roots, which suck up valuable soil minerals and "feed" them to the more shallow-rooting vines. They also prevent the growth of unwanted weeds and grasses.

The vineyard's other unusual feature is a wooden barrel set in the middle of the plantation. Open to the sky, it looks modest and even non-descript, but it's central to their viticulture, says Hayo. After it's filled with rainwater, it receives a variety of herbs and plants, plus Steiner's signature dish of cow dung matured in cow horns. Every few months, at special times in the lunar cycle, the water is "dynamised" by violent vortexing with a wooden paddle, and then sprayed onto the vines. The liquid is claimed to be such a powerful fertiliser that the vines grow strongly enough to withstand insect and fungal attacks. But Hayo admits that there's also some extra celestial assistance. "Our dynamised sprays create a sensitive relationship between the forces of the Earth and those of the Moon, Venus and Mercury, our nearest heavenly bodies," he says. "When the Moon descends, the Earth inhales, concentrating the growth forces on the soil beneath the vines."

Perhaps surprisingly, such mysticisms have not dissuaded other growers from following suit. In fact, a remarkable 1% of the world vineyards have now completely embraced biodymanics - from modest Spanish *viñedos* to top French *domaines*. In fact, the world's most expensive wines come from Domaine de la Romanée Conti, a Burgundy vineyard which went biodynamic in 2007.

A few kilometres away from Romanée Conti is the vineyard of an even earlier adopter, Madame Lalou Bize-Leroy. She's a passionate biodynamicist, with plaques showing the Signs of the Zodiac adorning her cellars: "The vines respond to the radiations from individual constellations", she says. But again, don't mock. Her wines are among the best Burgundies on the market, with experts searching for superlatives to describe them - hardly surprising when a single one of her bottles can cost as much as a small car ($35,000)

However, the question must be asked: while the health benefits of organic wine are obvious - in particular the absence of man-made pesticides, fungicides, herbicides etc.[258] - are there any extra benefits to be had from 'super-organic' biodynamics?

Certain that there would be a ready answer to the question (after all, health was Steiner's main motivation), I contacted Demeter, the Swiss-based HQ of the biodynamic movement. They seemed glad to help. "Please contact NW, our expert on the subject." But sadly, NW didn't reply, and neither did their two other suggested experts.

Fortunately, biodynamics is now growing so rapidly that there are other organisations rivalling Demeter for the top spot. One of these is Biodyvin, whose founder Olivier Humbrecht owns a flourishing group of small biodynamic vineyards stretching across 100 acres in Alsace. His annual crop of 27 different white wines score very highly among wine experts.

As a very committed biodynamicist, he's keen to establish the science behind his huge investment in the technique. So when I quizzed him on it, he knew exactly what I was after: "You want to know if biodynamics isn't just a hoax," he said bluntly.

Well, even if the word "hoax" is a bit strong - "wishful thinking" might have been kinder - it's on the right lines, and Olivier was able to steer me to a surprisingly large body of scientific research.

Biodynamics: the verdict

So now, dear reader, after my deep dive into scores of research papers on your behalf, how does biodynamics (bio) compare to straight organics (org)?

One clear difference is the cost to the grower: going org is already reckoned to cost 15% more than conventional viticulture, but going bio adds another 15%. The other financial problem is that grape yields can be up to 40% lower than on conventional vineyards. Hence the stonking bottle prices.*

As for the scientific evidence, Humbrecht is keen to point out that his own soil micro-organisms are ten times more plentiful now that he's gone bio than when purely org, and that his vines' mineral deficiencies are now at an end.

It's also clear that bio vineyards tend to be more biodiverse, with an abundance of wildlife.

But thereafter, sad to say, the extra benefits of bio appear to be patchy at best, as seen through the brutal lens of science.

For example in one experiment, four identical plots were chosen in a Californian Merlot vineyard for a six year head-to-head contest between bio and org. The results were a win for bio, but nothing spectacular. The major difference was that bio grapes had more dissolved sugars and polyphenols, but in only one season out of the six.[259]

---

* Although you can find some biodynamic wines at less than $15 a bottle

Furthermore, a very similar experiment was done in Germany, which again found that " no differences between the organic and the biodynamic treatment occurred."[260]

Next question, is there any difference in the quality of the wines themselves? Again sadly no, according to a review of the evidence, which reported that "the chemical and sensory properties of organic and biodynamic wines do not differ."[261]

It was the same story on a Sangiovese vineyard in Italy, where

> No significant difference [in wine contents] was shown among the samples coming from different wine-making practices.[262]

Indeed, one Italian study found that bio wines were actually inferior to org ones, reporting that

> Sangiovese wines from biodynamic production showed decreased alcohol content, decreased phenolic compounds, decreased wine colour, decreased total polymeric pigments and decreased tannin concentration.[263]

So, having drawn a bit of a blank with biodynamics itself, I reframed the question. Because their wines are much more costly to produce, if only for the extra care taken in growing them, are expensive wines intrinsically healthier?

For years, most experts in wines' health benefits have maintained that all wines are the same. Provided your bottle of cheap plonk contains the genuine liquid made from fermented grapes, they have said, it's just as health-promoting as the best Château de N'importe où Premier Cru.

But that's been questioned by recent research. In one study, 60 differently priced Italian red wines were compared. The findings confounded received medical opinion: the most expensive wines had the highest polyphenol contents (i.e. good news), and the plonks the lowest polyphenols and highest histamine levels (bad news).[264]

Incidentally, why are histamines bad news? They're one of a category of newly discovered natural chemicals called biogenic amines, which inevitably arise during the wine-making process. For most people, histamines aren't a problem, but for a significant minority of drinkers they cause headaches and even migraines.[265]

Interestingly, sulphites in wine tend to reduce histamine levels. So paradoxically, rather than causing headaches, sulphites might help prevent them.

Lunar Thuns

But back to biodynamics. Nearly a century after Steiner's death, one of his fans, a German agricultural smallholder called Maria Thun, came up with the interesting claim that the taste of wines differed on certain days according to the moon's path through the stellar constellations. She decided to publish her claims, specifying the best days in the year for drinking wine ("fruit" and "flower" days) and the worst ("root" and "leaf" days).[266]

Remarkably, Thun's book became an instant best-seller: people did indeed find that wines tasted either better or worse in line with her predictions. Exciting stuff. News travelled fast through the intimate world of wine, and soon got taken up by commerce. When British supermarkets launched new lines in wines, their PR people reportedly took care to invite journalists to wine-tastings only on Thun's favourable days.

But was there anything to it, or was it all a hoax? Only recently has the world of science investigated.

In 2016, Dr Wendy Parr and her team at the Department of Wine, Food and Molecular Biosciences at Lincoln University, New Zealand assembled a group of 19 wine experts and put them to the test. Would they blind-judge a high quality Pinot Noir differently according to Thun's almanac?

The answer was a resounding no. Although - perhaps surprisingly - the experts' assessments did differ from day to day, there was zero connection with leaf, flower, root or fruit days....nor indeed with any lunar cycle or even weather pattern.[267]

Summary

Organic wines tend to be higher quality than conventionally produced ones, containing fewer sulphites (in the USA) and zero pesticide residues.

It's largely a myth that sulphites are unhealthy - except for a tiny minority of drinkers.

There is no evidence that biodynamic viticulture produces better wines than organic husbandry.

13

Alcohol-free Wine

Suppose – never mind whether it could be chemically possible, please God not – that a totally non-alcoholic wine could be invented that possessed all the appeal to the senses that alcoholic varieties offer. Do you honestly believe that connoisseurs and ordinary wine-drinkers alike would embrace the product?[268]

That powerful *cri de coeur* came from the pen of Matthew Parris, columnist for *The Times* of London and *Spectator* magazine. When he wrote that in 2017, he must have imagined that whole idea of alcohol-free wines was dystopian science fiction. But little did he know that, for over a decade, chemists had been plotting how to suck the alcohol out of wine. Indeed, shortly after Parris' piece, his nightmare actually came true. Tentatively at first, British supermarkets began offering denatured wine under 'own label' brands, keen to appear to be offering healthy alternatives to the real thing.

Remarkably, this has now been taken up by wine-growers across the world. Even French viticulturalists have succumbed - although the whole idea must have almost literally stuck in their throats. After all, France is the very country whose workaday culture once demanded a restorative wine-drenched lunch before an afternoon nap. And these were substantial amounts. Soldiers in the WW1 trenches received a daily ration of 2 litres of red wine (yes, nearly three standard-sized bottles of wine) a day. After the war, even lowly workers in Parisian restaurants were offered the same 2 litre daily allowance, George Orwell tells us.[269]

Less than a century later, however, wine drinking in France has now declined to a level that would have appalled those French low-life denizens. The latest estimate is that the average Frenchman now drinks barely 40 litres of wine in a whole *year*, and over a third of the populace never touches a drop - a profound cultural revolution ripe for exploitation by the zero or low alcohol wine market.

But France is still a minnow: the big fish in the fake wine sea are mainly anglophone countries. Wine drinkers in North America appear to be the most enthusiastic, with a take-up growth rate of 8% year on year, say industry insiders.

Why the growing switch from real wines to denatured ones?

Well, according to surveys, the main one is practical: being able to drive home after dinner parties. Very responsible, very middle-class.

But the reasons go much deeper. First, a cultural revolution in attitudes to getting slammed - particularly among the professional classes, such as journalists and lawyers (but perhaps not politicians). For example, when I was a BBC producer, I well remember liquid lunches in the well-stocked bars kindly provided by the management in most BBC premises (Lord alone knows how we got any work done in the afternoons). But of course, those bars are now pretty empty at lunchtimes, as are the pubs of Fleet Street, the one-time home of British newspapers.

The second driver of the zero alcohol push is some very effective PR by a consortium of alcohol 'charities'. Mainly British, with euphemistic names such as Alcohol Concern and Alcohol Change, in 2013 these quasi-prohibitionist bodies invented Dry January - an exhortation to go a whole month without downing a molecule of alcohol. Timed to harness the guilt of an excessively boozy Christmas and its attendant hangovers, Dry January * has rapidly become a popular penance for the chattering classes, keen to virtue-signal their

---

* Now with four clones: "Sober Spring", "Sober September", "Sober October" and "Alcoholfree 40" (during the Christian Lent)

abstinence - or perhaps to challenge their ability to spend a whole month 'on the wagon'.

But the major driver of the anti-booze movement is undoubtedly the attitude of the authorities and their implied condemnation of alcohol by relentlessly reducing the officially 'safe' levels of drinking (see chapter 14).

One gets the feeling that we are all being softened up to hear that there is no safe level of drinking at all. Indeed, this has already happened in the case of cancer.

> From the point of view of cancer prevention, the best level of alcohol consumption is zero

says the World Cancer Research Foundation.[270]

On the other hand, as chapter 2 has already shown, that blanket condemnation of alcohol should not apply to wine, with wine drinkers overall having a lower cancer risk than non-drinkers - and indeed a reduced risk of heart disease, diabetes, dementia etc. etc.

So the question to be answered is this: given the privileged position of wine, are there any health advantages to drinking alcohol-free versions of the liquid?

Here goes another deep dive…

Real v. Alcohol-free wines: the health evidence

First off, I must declare an interest. While I cannot distinguish between the taste of alcohol-free lagers and real ones, much enjoying either at sunny lunchtimes, I cannot say the same for fake wines at dinner. For some reason, they don't seem to combine with food with the same richness as the real thing. Quite simply, alcohol-free wine is not to my taste. So my gut feeling - literally - is that the real thing must be better.

But, as you will doubtless have deduced by now, this book is uniquely led by the medical evidence, not by my personal opinion.

The problem is that alcohol-free wines haven't been around long enough to have amassed enough epidemiological data to offer a definitive judgement on my wholly unscientific gut feeling. By definition, there can be no research comparing the long-term benefits of proper wine and alcohol-free wine (for brevity, I will refer to the former as "real wine" and the latter "fake wine").

However, there have been some short-term clinical studies which paradoxically may be more useful. Simply put, healthy human volunteers (mainly young men, short of a penny or two, and with time on their hands) have been brought into laboratories to compare their various bodily functions after consuming real and fake wines. Modern technology makes this both easy and instructive, as the data obtained provide solid evidence of harm or benefit, by measuring so-called bodily "biomarkers".

Much of this research has been carried out in two countries at opposite ends of Europe: Spain and Finland.

One of the first studies was at Finland's Turku University where doctors measured blood flow through the heart. They found a clear difference between real and fake wine, with the real stuff increasing the men's "coronary flow velocity reserve" (CFVR). There's no doubt whatever that a good CFVR is a very healthy outcome.[271]

Interestingly, the Finns found that alcohol on its own does not increase CFVR, implying that there's a health-promoting synergy between real wine's ingredients of polyphenols and alcohol. In other words, it would seem that grape juice needs to be fermented to have any CFVR benefit.

A second Finnish study found that "high doses" of real wine inhibit blood clotting, while alcohol itself and fake wine do not.[272] Now is that good or bad news? The Finns say it's bad news because blood which won't clot properly is a risk factor for heart disease. Fair enough, but on the other hand, if your blood doesn't clot easily, it means it's been thinned, thus reducing the risk of an ischemic stroke and high blood pressure. Indeed, many heart disease patients are often prescribed blood-thinning drugs called vasodilators. And you don't have to be a patient to benefit from vasodilation. For

110

example, if you were drinking real wine during the Covid crisis, you might have been protected against the blood clots associated with both the illness and the vaccines.

In summary, the Finns' research findings are pretty clear that real wine has far more health benefits than fake wine.

Australian dieticians have also investigated the fake wine health question on post-menopausal women prone to high levels of harmful cholesterol. For six weeks the women were asked to drink either half a bottle of fake or real wine a day, after which they were swapped around in what's called a Crossover Trial. At the end of each six week session, their cholesterol levels were tested. Fake wine was found to have no effect whatever, but real wine increased beneficial (HDL) cholesterol and reduced harmful (LDL) cholesterol. [273]

Similar human guinea-pig tests have been done in the USA, where muscadine red wine was compared to muscadine grape juice, finding that:

> Consumption of wine, but not grape juice, significantly increased antioxidant capacity and resulted in beneficial changes to blood vessels.[274]

In 2009 German diabetes experts reported on the results of a clinical trial which again pitched real and fake wines head to head. They knew that real wine reduced the risk of diabetes, but they wanted to see if fake wine would do just as well. The biomarker they tested was adinopectin, a valuable protein known to reduce the risk of diabetes, arterial disease and obesity. However, once again, fake wine failed the test, having "no substantial effect on adiponectin concentrations", whereas real wine did.[275]

What's the Spanish verdict? Spain's major alcohol and health research centre is at the University of Barcelona where Professor Ramon Estruch, one of the country's leading alcohol experts, runs the Institut d'Investigacions Biomèdiques. Over the last twenty years, he and his research team have conducted a host of clinical trials on alcoholic drinks - probably the most anywhere in the world.

Estruch's laboratory bristles with high-tech analytical hardware, generating sophisticated measurements of health biomarkers in samples of bodily fluids. In chapter 3, we saw how his research on the body's beneficial reactions to both spirits and wine offers incontrovertible evidence to support the real-world findings that drinkers have less heart disease than non-drinkers.[276]

As soon as alcohol-free wines began to take off, Estruch was keen to discover how much better - or worse - they might be for drinkers' health. So he set about comparing real and fake wines in clinical trials, mimicking the ones often used in the pharmaceutical industry. In an early trial, he asked 70 healthy adult volunteers to alternate between real and fake wines in 4 week periods, to see what effects each had on the body. They were given nearly half a bottle of wine to drink per day with meals.

It wasn't plain sailing, however, as many of his human guinea pigs could barely tolerate the taste of fake wine, with two of them actually refusing to drink it. Still, those who stomached it provided some useful information.

First, the blood data showed there was no difference between real and fake wine in terms of glucose metabolism, with each being equally beneficial.[277]

That's an important finding, as efficient glucose metabolism decreases the risk of diabetes and obesity. So full marks to both real and fake wine for that.

But not for a substance in the blood called lipoprotein (a). Here, there was a significant difference, with real wine showing much lower levels than fake wine. What do higher lp(a) levels mean health-wise? Sadly for fake wine drinkers, it's bad news, as lp(a) is a risk factor for atherosclerosis (furred-up arteries), coronary heart disease and stroke.[278] 1 in 6 of us have high lp(a) levels, so the study suggests that a significant proportion of the population could benefit from drinking real wine rather than the fake stuff.

But surely there must be some be benefit from fake wine, Estruch told himself. One obvious area is the simple one of high blood pressure, as it's been known for over a century that excessive drinking can raise it fairly substantially.[279]

Estruch's hunch was right.

In another 3 month clinical trial, he found that, although moderate amounts of both real and fake wine reduced blood pressure, the latter reduced it slightly more - but only by a "modest" amount, he says.[280]

Estruch's team have also compared real and fake wine's effect on gut bacteria, the microbiome discussed in chapter 8. Again, by clinically testing volunteers, they found a significant difference in gut health - again in real wine's favour:

> The diversity of the fecal microbiota was higher after the red wine dosing period. We found a significant increase in the *Proteobacteria, Firmicutes*, and *Bacteroidetes* phyla, but not after the de-alcoholized red wine period. Moreover, after the red wine period, there was an important decrease in the *Clostridium* genera and *Clostridium histolyticum* group. [281]

In layman's language: compared to fake wine, real wine improves the diversity of gut bacteria, as well as increasing beneficial bacteria and reducing harmful bacteria.

So far therefore, in the Health Stakes horse race, the real wine stallion is already many lengths ahead of his gelding rival.

But the real wine's lead is about to open up even further, because of Hydroxytyrosol[HT]

Back in chapter 11, you may remember reading that HT is a recently discovered constituent of both wine and olive oil, and is now thought to be a key explanation for the health benefits of a Mediterranean diet. In fact, wine may be even more important than olive oil, because laboratory tests have shown that wine produces 40% more HT in the body than olive oil.[282]

In 2015 another Spanish research team led by Professor Rafael de la Torre asked the key question in this chapter: vis-à-vis HT, is fake wine as health-promoting as real wine?

Once again, the answer was sought from human guinea pigs. "28 healthy male subjects" aged about 26 were given a small glass of real and fake wine, in two suitably spaced sessions. At the end of each session their urine was tested for the presence of HT. The results were astonishing: in these men's bodies, real wine produced more than twice the amount of HT than fake wine.[283]

On the face of it, however, this is puzzling. After all, the antioxidant polyphenols in both real and fake wine are exactly the same, so how can the presence of alcohol, which is not itself an antioxidant, increase the antioxidant value of real wine?

De la Torre says the answer lies in dopamine, a chemical which our bodies naturally produce when we feel pleasure. Lying in the sun, having sex, listening to music, all produce dopamine - and so does drinking alcohol, probably due to its relaxing effect. OK, but so what? De la Torre's crucial discovery has been that dopamine forms a chemical bond with an ingredient in wine called tyrosol, resulting in the actual manufacture of HT within the body.[284]

This is a stunning finding: that the alcohol in real wine contributes to its health benefits by its beneficial effects on mood.

Put simply, getting gently squiffy is good for your health.

In fact, alcohol's effects as a de-stressor are only now beginning to be studied. Medics at Massachusetts General Hospital have found that drinking produces less "stress signalling" in the amygdala, the part of the brain that regulates fear responses. This could help reduce blood pressure and risk of stroke and heart attack, particularly in the chronically stressed, say the researchers.[285]

So what's the expert verdict on real v. fake wines? This was Professor Estruch's pithy answer to my question:

> My conclusion is that the beneficial effects of wine are due to its alcohol and polyphenol components. Apart from possible effects on blood pressure, regular wine is 'better' than de-alcoholised wine since it combines the beneficial effects of alcohol and polyphenols.[286]

114

There are only a very few narrow categories of people who shouldn't drink real wine, says Estruch:

> Pregnant mothers, the underage, people on certain medications or with pre-existing conditions (e.g. liver disease), or holding religious beliefs (e.g. Muslims).

Why is fake wine so unappealing?

Here's a quote from an Italian consumer survey:

> Alcohol-free wines generate a significant aversion in consumers. Our data show that only 10% of [people] are willing to buy de-alcoholised wine.[287]

One reason for consumer distaste may be that removing the alcohol from wine needs a substantial amount of processing. A variety of techniques are used: centrifugation, reverse osmosis, vacuum steam distillation, osmotic transport, spinning-cone column, thin-film evaporation under reduced pressure, and thermal gradient process. The resulting liquid is little more than a "syrup", say the Italians. To attempt to restore it to a semblance of wine, bottlers add water, concentrated must, gum arabic, deacidifiers, clarifiers, grape juice, and grape juice concentrate.

The resultant product in your glass would appear to be the wine equivalent of ultra-processed food - a commodity increasingly shown to be harmful to health.

Summary

Real wine is better for your health than alcohol-free wine, as alcohol and wine's natural ingredients appear to act synergistically. Real wine is a better vasodilator, thus improving blood flow; it makes for a healthier gut, prevents diabetes and atherosclerosis, reduces heart disease risk and has higher levels of hydroxytyrosol, a potent antioxidant. It also reduces stress.

14

Dis- Mis- and Mal- Information

Opinion polls show that people are confused about alcohol and health - and wine in particular. Friends who know I have written about alcohol often complain that the newspapers are full of contradictory stories about the subject. One week we're told that drinking can be good for you, the next that you'll die a grisly death if you touch a single drop. For example, within the space of a couple of weeks in July 2021, these two headlines appeared : "New study links moderate alcohol use with higher cancer risk."[288] and "A tipple a day cuts death risk, study shows."[289]

This is not at all unusual. Stretching back years, there's been a consistent pattern of conflicting 'alcohol and health' press stories. One day drinking is harmful, another it's beneficial. That's not only confusing, but it sounds bonkers. After all, with tobacco, lighting up is always bad news for your health. But not with drinking. Why?

The most obvious reason could be that behind the 'good news about booze' stories are naked commercial interests. For example in the past, the tobacco industry has routinely funded scientific research which downplayed the risks of smoking. The food industry has also consistently suborned nutritional science – and still does.[290]

Food additives are a good example: almost all the studies which find they are harmless have been funded by the additive industry.[291]

An even more notorious example is with sugar. A recent investigation found that 50 years ago the sugar industry "sponsored a research program that successfully cast doubt about the hazards of sucrose, while promoting fat as the dietary culprit in heart disease." [292] Such blatant corruption of academic research by industry bribery has been directly responsible for the developed world's greatest chronic health crisis: the obesity pandemic. Years of Big Food dollars funnelled to US universities - even to such august places as Harvard - have ensured that research findings have been routinely skewed to demonstrate that overweight is caused not by high-carbohydrate but by high-fat diets. Hence the heavy promotion of low-fat foods, with disastrous consequences for health.

So it would be an obvious move by the alcohol industry to follow suit, by bribing alcohol researchers to promote alcohol's health benefits. Indeed, this is a charge often levelled by the anti-alcohol brigade. But is it true?

Broadly, no. Although there are instances of the industry funding meta-analyses (pull-togethers of the existing evidence), a review of those studies' outcomes shows no bias in the findings. [293] More importantly, the alcohol industry doesn't fund any original research. Indeed, a recent attempt to solicit industry cash for a major new research study provoked such an outcry that the proposal – again Harvard-based - never got off the ground. [294]

The fact is that, although there are literally hundreds of 'alcohol and health' studies published every year - some at great expense - almost all are funded by government health authorities, working mainly through universities and clinical research groups.

On the other hand, bias and corruption isn't a one-way street: in the case of alcohol, it can be used either to promote drinking or oppose it. And latterly there's been a huge increase in oppositional propaganda - much of it, if not corrupt, deliberately misleading. Its main target has been the subject of this book: namely, the very notion that drinking can be good for you.

Lying about the evidence

Covering up alcohol's health benefits goes back a long way. One of the first instances occurred in the early 1950s, at the end of a study on the inhabitants of Framingham, a small town in Massachusetts. The town had been chosen as the location for a huge US government-funded research program on lifestyle and health. Because heart disease was such a killer, one of the first things they wanted to know was how to prevent it. So a team of top Harvard researchers was employed to dig deep into the inhabitants' health and lifestyle records to see if they could detect any lifestyle patterns.

Lo and behold, one thing that stood out a mile was that alcohol drinkers had less heart disease than non-drinkers, and the research team wrote up the findings accordingly. But when they submitted them to their government paymasters, they got seriously torn off a strip. They were instructed to:

> Remove all references to alcohol. An article which openly invites the encouragement of drinking with the implication of preventing CHD [heart disease] would be scientifically misleading and socially undesirable in view of the major problem of alcoholism that already exists in this country. If you must say something about alcohol, say it has no effect.

But the Harvard researchers refused to capitulate. Rather than lie, they kept quiet about their findings, and waited for their paymasters to move on... finally publishing their heretical evidence over a decade later.[295]

Such blatant censorship appears to be a thing of the past, but the more recent deceptions are much more insidious, because they often come with well orchestrated anti-alcohol PR, ensuring dramatic headlines.

For example, in 2018 a Cambridge University research team published the pooled findings from over 80 studies, involving nearly 600,000 drinkers, which claimed to have overturned half a century of research at a stroke.[296] "(Our) findings challenge the widely held belief that moderate drinking is beneficial to cardiovascular health," trumpeted the accompanying press release. The study received huge publicity, creating headlines such as "drinking five glasses of wine a week can take years off your life," and "drinking is as harmful as smoking."

However, this turned out to be nonsense: the researchers had found nothing of the sort. Data sleuths (myself included) soon discovered the truth. Buried deep in the Cambridge study's voluminous published appendix were the raw figures which, far from challenging the idea that drinking doesn't benefit cardiovascular health, unequivocally confirmed it, with the data showing a clear reduction in heart disease risk at moderate alcohol intakes. They demonstrated that, compared to lifetime non-drinkers, people who drank between 18 and 28 grams of alcohol a day (one to two glasses of wine) were found to have a 40 per cent reduction in "all cardiovascular events" (i.e. deaths from or symptoms of heart and circulatory disease). Above that level of intake, the benefit was found to tail off, but there was still a 20 per cent reduction even at an intake of 78 grams (a whole bottle of wine) a day.

In other words, the Cambridge researchers had found cardiovascular health benefits at low, moderate and high alcohol intakes. The press release was an outright lie.

I emailed the principal author (one of a ludicrously high number of 130 named authors, some quite eminent) of the paper about this blatant contradiction between the press release and the study's actual data, but received no answer. And yet that paper is still widely cited* as evidence for alcohol's lack of health benefits - probably because it has a Cantabrigian provenance.

Another anti-alcohol ruse is to ignore data which don't fit the prohibitionist narrative. The most blatant example of this censorship came from a team at Canada's Center for Addictions Research. In 2016, they published what was they claimed was a meta-analysis of moderate drinkers' mortality rates, announcing in the summary that the evidence was too

---

* in fact, cited over 1000 times

weak to be anything but "skeptical" about alcohol's health benefits. Once again, one had to be a data sleuth to discover in the small print that the Canadians' downbeat conclusion was based on an assessment of only 6 studies, carefully chosen from a grand total of 2662 studies on drinkers' mortality rates.[297] Clearly, cherry-picking such an infinitesimal fraction of the available evidence is meaningless, and tantamount to pseudoscience. That the paper should ever have been published is deplorable, but once again it's routinely cited as evidence for alcohol's lack of health benefits.

Another anti-alcohol PR trick involves wine itself. Research scientists are hungry for publicity, so they know that attacking wine drinking - and thus putting the frighteners on the chattering classes and their favourite tipple - will generate headlines. This tactic was clearly behind the announcement of the results of an Oxford University study[298] in 2022, which *The Times* reported as: "5 glasses of wine a week can cause premature ageing".[299] Scary stuff.

I want to examine this story in some detail, as it's a classic example of how journalism via press release is employed to reinforce the anti-alcohol narrative.

There were five reasons why *The Times* got it wrong.

First, the study wasn't about wine itself, but alcohol in general. Second, the Oxford researchers had merely found that drinkers had shorter telomeres than non-drinkers. What are telomeres? They're microscopic additions on the end of chromosomes, whose length is believed to be a marker for longevity. However, the whole issue of telomeres and longevity is "controversial"[300], so firm conclusions are inherently hard to justify. Third, the study results had already been challenged by Harvard scientists who had found no such connection.[301] Fourth, a study specifically on wine and longevity had contradicted Oxford, finding that "moderate red wine consumption increases the expression of key longevity-related genes"[302]. Finally, another study had found that "adherence to the Mediterranean diet (of which red wine is a key component) is associated with longer telomeres."[303]

120

So *The Times* story was not worth the paper it was printed on. But of course, that judgment is grossly unfair: journalists have neither the time nor expertise to question PR handouts - particularly ones from prestigious institutions. And such institutions are themselves disinclined to present a rounded picture of the available evidence, for fear of blunting the PR value of their latest 'shock-horror' findings.

Perhaps the most egregious example of 'demonise wine at all costs' was a 2019 paper subtitled: "How many cigarettes are there in a bottle of wine?"[304] - a bizarre rhetorical question clearly designed to lead the reader to conclude that wine is as harmful as tobacco. This was not an original study, but an assessment of the existing published evidence. But here's the extraordinary, barely credible fact. Although there were at the time over 10,000 studies on wine and health, the authors of this study cited *not a single one* as evidence.

How can a scientific paper which claims that drinking wine is as unhealthy as smoking possibly be published, let alone taken seriously, if it fails to provide a scrap of evidence? How can it pass the peer-review process - the very system designed to prevent pseudoscience from seeing the light of day? The answer is simple: journals will publish any nonsense provided it fits the prevailing semi-Prohibitionist narrative.

Another increasingly favoured ruse is to conduct studies in the Far East. As chapter 6 showed, Asians and Mongoloids tend to have poorly protective alcohol dehydrogenase enzymes, making them more susceptible to the toxic effects of acetaldehyde, the first breakdown product of alcohol. One such study was published in 2019[305] to lurid headlines: "Even one drink a day increases stroke risk," screamed the press.

One of the authors was even quoted as saying: "The alcohol industry should be regulated in a similar way to the tobacco industry."

At first sight, the study looked impressive: a decade-long comparison of the health data from half a million people – some drinkers, some non-drinkers.

But here comes the problem: the half million people were Chinese - all handicapped by their genetically weak protective enzymes. And the study's difficulties don't end there. The Chinese have an unusual drinking culture: most Chinese drinkers prefer very strong spirits, often consumed in a binge-drinking environment.

Nevertheless, the study reported remarkably few ill effects from drinking. For example, drinkers' risk of having a heart attack was no different from that of non-drinkers. Their only significant health difference was in the two types of stroke: a 58 percent increased risk for hemorrhagic stroke (where a blood vessel bursts in the brain), and 27 percent for ischemic stroke (where blood flow is blocked or interrupted).

Those were the figures for the heaviest drinkers, but they are clinically meaningless. All they show is that Chinese drinkers have less than twice the extra risk of a stroke (by comparison, smokers have up to 25 times the extra risk of lung cancer). The PR hooha surrounding the study was sheer hype.

The final disinformation tactic is simply to lie. The latest example of this is in Canada, whose authorities now claim that "even very small amounts of alcohol can be harmful to people's health and well-being"[306] - a blatant deceit, because the truth is the direct reverse, as this book has amply shown.

The Canadians appear to be classic totalitarians, their playbook straight out of Nazi Germany. In 1928, propaganda minister Joseph Goebbels tellingly said this:

> Propaganda is not supposed to be...theoretically correct. Its point...is to persuade people of what we think right.[307]

21st Century "Prohibition"

I put the P-word in quotes, because not even the most fanatical anti-alcohol activist is foolish enough to push for an outright alcohol ban - but we're getting close to a *de facto* one. The primary tactic has been to use increasingly draconian official national drinking 'guidelines'.

Astonishingly, alcohol guidelines are not much more than half a century old, and were originally "plucked out of the air", as one committee member later confessed. The first time real science was deployed to establish national guidelines was in 1995, when a committee of British civil servants did an in-depth investigation of the medical evidence for alcohol's health pros and cons, and came up with a daily maximum of 4 'units' a day for men, and half that for women. 4 UK units roughly equals 3 gins, one and a half pints of beer, and slightly over a third of a bottle of wine. As it happens, that figure was an extremely enlightened recommendation, because 4 units corresponds to what the data then showed would *maximise* alcohol's overall health benefits, while minimising its harms.

Other countries tended to follow Britain's liberal lead - even the USA, the very birthplace of Prohibition. As recently as 2015, the US Government-appointed scientists on the Dietary Guidelines Advisory Committee were writing (my emphases):

> *The U.S. population should be encouraged and guided to consume dietary patterns that are* rich in vegetables, fruits, whole grains, seafood, legumes, and nuts; *moderate in* low- and non-fat dairy products and *alcohol* (among adults); lower in red and processed meat; and low in sugar-sweetened foods and beverages and refined grains.... *Moderate alcohol intake can be a component of a healthy diet.*[308]

However, things began to change markedly the very next year, with what appeared to be a takeover of the international medical establishment by the prohibitionist lobby. Pressure was put on politicians drastically to reduce the alcohol guidelines, on the pretext that "there is no safe level of drinking", and even that "the idea that drinking a glass of red wine a day is good for you is an old wives' tale" - a pathetic little fabrication from none other than England's Chief Medical Officer.[309]

But the medical authorities' most serious claim was that there was new evidence of increased cancer risk at very low intakes, announcing:

> There is no level of regular drinking that can be considered as completely safe in relation to some cancers.[310]

However, in order to arrive at this verdict, it was necessary to employ some serious jiggery-pokery. This was achieved by the UK medical authorities commissioning a private assessment of the existing evidence from Sheffield University, resulting in a 'behind closed doors' report which avoided the external peer-review process, and so had no independent scrutiny. Furthermore, thanks to some Freedom of Information ferreting by British journalist Christopher Snowdon, we now know that the university's initial report was rejected by the British medical authorities as being too favourable to alcohol. Pressure was then applied on the university to manipulate the evidence to exaggerate alcohol's health hazards and downgrade its benefits.[311]

For example, one of the studies Sheffield would doubtless have been required to ignore was a 2013 research paper entitled "Alcohol drinking and all-cancer mortality". This huge survey of the international medical evidence found that, far from causing cancer at low intakes, alcohol in fact does the reverse, concluding:

> (Our) meta-analysis confirms the health hazards of heavy drinking and the benefits of light drinking.[312]

The study showed that low alcohol intakes (under 12.5 grams a day) reduce cancer risk, and that increased risk only begins to kick in at about 50 grams of alcohol a day (2.5 pints of beer, a few gins/whiskies, 2/3rds of a bottle of wine), and then only modestly.

The Guidelines

Nevertheless, whether by deceit or not, the prohibitionists won the day, and for whatever reason - follow the crowd, hairshirtism, authoritarianism - the overwhelming majority of medical authorities across the world followed the British example, sometimes reducing their drinking limits to ludicrously low levels. For example, Holland and Canada have now slashed their guidelines to almost zero.

This is what the various national guidelines are in 2023, compared to an arbitrary date in the recent past:

History of alcohol guidelines (for men)*		
Grams of alcohol per day One bottle of wine contains about 80 grams		
	2006	*2023*
Australia	40	14
Austria	24	24
Canada	27	4
Finland	23.5	20
France	None	20
Hong Kong	30	20
Ireland	30	24
Italy	36	24
Japan	40	20
Netherlands	30	10
New Zealand	30	21
Spain	30	40
Switzerland	24	19
UK	32	16
USA	56	28

*For women's intakes, most countries halve men's daily rates

Summary

Is medical research on alcohol corrupted by vested interests? The alcohol industry appears to be blameless, but not the 'charitable' anti-alcohol sector. It has successfully pressurised medical authorities to reduce the recommended limits on drinking, so that today's 'guidelines' are significantly lower than before, largely on the basis of manipulated evidence.

15

FAQs

Q. If wine is so good for you, why has research found that there is a limit to how much wine you can drink for optimum health?

A. Simple: it's the alcohol in wine that's the problem.

For those of us fortunate enough to enjoy a few glasses a day, it's perhaps worth reminding ourselves just how poisonous alcohol really is. Think of what alcohol is used for when it's not flowing down our throats.

Alcohol (and its identical twin, ethanol) is an industrial chemical, being used both as a powerful solvent and as an additive to petrol – indeed, cars will run entirely on ethanol.

Alcohol is also a potent disinfectant, routinely used by hospitals as a hand-cleanser to prevent infection. To borrow the familiar script of lavatory cleaner commercials, alcohol kills 99.9% of germs stone dead. So it's as vicious as bleach.

It's also a powerful preservative. If you want to keep a corpse (or any parts thereof) from rotting, immerse it in alcohol. It will last for ever. Only formalin will do as good a job.

So alcohol is seriously cytotoxic – it kills living cells.

That's why the body has developed the two alcohol-detoxifying enzymes ADH and ALDH, which are particularly potent in people of European descent. Nevertheless the enzymes aren't miracle workers. If they're overwhelmed by alcohol, they'll fail. Because this creates a potentially dangerous situation, the body has a reserve back-up system with a long scientific name: the Microsomal Ethanol Oxidising System. First discovered in the 1970s, MEOS is an emergency rescue system in the liver which neutralises the excess alcohol by breaking down its molecules; it kicks in after "chronic heavy alcohol consumption", says the experimental evidence.[313]

But there's a problem. While MEOS prevents you from being killed by excess alcohol, the breakdown products can be nasty. The main one is the potentially cancer-causing acetaldehyde which, unlike in normal alcohol metabolism, doesn't get quickly turned into harmless acetic acid. Other metabolites are Reactive Oxygen Species. These are mildly carcinogenic too, but their main disadvantage is that they whizz around the body destroying valuable nutrients - thus wiping out any benefits from wine's polyphenols.

That's a sciency explanation for why it's important to keep one's wine intake within sensible (i.e not insensible!) limits.

Q I can't promise to be a sensible drinker, so how can I protect myself against alcohol's nastier side-effects?

A. One major health consequence of excessive drinking is that the body becomes depleted of folate (Vitamin B9). As chapter 2 showed, a folate deficiency can increase the risk of certain types of cancer, and it can cause liver disease too.[314] So it would make sense to pop a daily folate supplement.

However, note that folate is often sold as folic acid, which although chemically very similar to natural folate, is not as bioavailable as folate itself,[315] which is derived from plants. How much does one need? The evidence indicates that drinkers require a minimum of 400 micrograms a day for protection against alcohol-related diseases. For example, a study of Australian women who drank the equivalent of 3 to 4 gins a day, had roughly twice the risk of breast cancer at low folate intakes, but that plummeted to 23% *less risk* if they were taking 400 mcgs of folate per day.[316] In other words, adequate folate can drastically reduce women's overall risk of breast cancer if they drink.

Another useful substance to mitigate the effects of heavy drinking is N-Acetylcysteine. This amino acid is a very powerful antioxidant which reduces inflammation, fights free radicals and reduces liver damage in experimental animals fed alcohol. [317] There's evidence that it can reduce alcohol cravings, too.[318] A typical dose is 600 mg per day.

Cravings can also be reduced by taking a gram a day of another amino acid, Acetyl-L-Carnitine.[319]

Q Which wine varieties have the most polyphenols?

A. There's no simple answer, as much depends on the grapes' growing conditions. For example, wines produced from grapes grown at high altitude will intrinsically have more polyphenols, because the vines will have had to generate more polyphenols to protect themselves from solar radiation. Vine husbandry and grape juice refining methods will also greatly affect polyphenol levels.

One thing is certain, however: red wine has far more than white. Assays show red contains between 1.8 and 3 grams of polyphenols per litre, while white lags way behind at one-sixth of those figures.[320]

Because of the effects of different growing conditions, it's difficult to decide which individual varietals score highest in terms of polyphenol content. As a rough guide, the darker the red wine, the more polyphenols. That rule of thumb tends to make Cabernet Sauvignon, Pinot Noir, Primitivo and Cannonau among the top scorers.

Q. What time of day is it best to drink?

A. In the evening with dinner. Why?

For two partly related reasons.

First, drinking with meals has been repeatedly shown to be the healthiest way to imbibe.[321] That's because food slows down the flow of alcohol into the bloodstream, while retaining wine's healthy polyphenols.

For example, a Spanish survey of nearly 20,000 people convincingly showed that people with a typical Mediterranean lifestyle (Med diet, red wine with meals, no binge drinking, low spirits intake) had half the risk of premature mortality of those who shunned the Med lifestyle, of which wine drinking is a major component.[322]

Reason no 2. is that evenings are when the alcohol detoxifying enzymes are at their most potent. Like the sleep/wake cycle and many other bodily functions, alcohol dehydrogenase enzymes operate on a roughly 24 hour circadian (Latin: *circa*=about, *dies*=day) schedule. Broadly speaking, the enzymes are least effective in the morning, but gradually get stronger through the day, reaching peak strength between 6pm and 8pm.[323]

This may explain why alcoholics often start drinking in the morning, as that time of day gives them the biggest hit from alcohol. It also explains why ordinary drinkers tend to find lunch-time drinking, although pleasurable enough at the time, can make them feel a bit seedy for the rest of the day.

Interestingly, alcohol craving has also been found to have a circadian cycle - lowest in the morning and highest in the evening,[324] thus exactly matching the enzyme activity. It's as if Mother Nature is deliberately nudging us to imbibe at times of the day when we're most likely to benefit from wine's contents, without the unhealthy consequences of ingesting too much alcohol. Clever!

Q I love my wine, but how can I avoid becoming an alcoholic?

A. The good news is that, if you're a wine drinker, your risk of alcoholism is far lower than with any other type of booze. The Danes, who spend gazillions of Kroner on alcohol research, are pretty clear on this,[325] as are the Canadians.[326]

The main reason is almost certainly the so-called "pattern of drinking" - the cultural norms, such as drinking with meals, which surround having a few glasses of wine. Also, unlike beer drinkers, wine drinkers generally don't binge drink, despite wine's higher level of alcohol content.

The other issue is how to define alcoholism. Alcohol's opponents often like to use the term "alcohol use disorder", trying to lump heavy drinking in with alcoholism, in order to artificially inflate the apparent problem.

But these are not at all the same animal, as acknowledged by as sober an institution as America's Center for Disease Control. "About 9 of 10 adult excessive drinkers [do] not meet the diagnostic criteria for alcohol dependence", says a major CDC survey.[327]

So it would appear that only 10% of heavy drinkers become alcoholics.

That's puzzling. If alcohol is truly an addictive substance, why don't 100% of drinkers fall into the deep dark pit of alcoholism? Most researchers shrug their shoulders, blaming 'genetics', but without much supporting evidence.

The most intriguing explanation blames the alcoholic's childhood. In 2004 Dr Vincent Felitti of Kaiser Permanente in San Diego made a breakthrough discovery linking alcoholism to "adverse childhood experiences" [ACEs].[328]

He found that the more ACEs someone had, the higher their risk of becoming an alcoholic - even as much as 50 years later.

These were Felliti's ACE categories:
1. recurrent and severe physical abuse
2. recurrent and severe emotional abuse
3. contact sexual abuse
4. Growing up in a household with:
   a   an alcoholic or drug-user
   b   a member being imprisoned
   c   a mentally ill, chronically depressed, or institutionalised member
   d   the mother being treated violently
   e   both biological parents being absent

Felitti employed a simple scoring system: one point for each ACE in someone's background. The chart of what he found is truly dramatic, not least because it looks remarkably like a dose response to a medication:

ACE Score vs. Adult Alcoholism

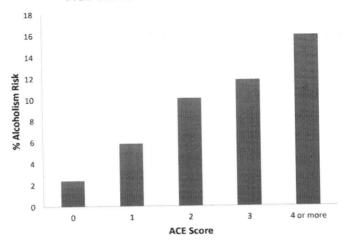

Derived from: Felitti VJ. The Origins of Addiction: Evidence from the Adverse Childhood Experiences Study, 2004

But of course, in this case it's not a response to a medication, but to a poison – a mental poison. Increase the ACE 'dose', and the risk of becoming an alcoholic rises proportionately. Not much of a surprise perhaps. After all, alcohol is a powerful mood-altering substance, so it may well act like a mental painkiller. By the way, Felliti's bombshell discovery has since been confirmed by researchers in Slovakia.[329]

"This psychodynamic explanation of alcoholism is obvious", he says, "but it's sometimes rejected in favour of a proposed genetic causality".

Clearly, alcoholics with ACE backgrounds need psychotherapy. For the rest of us with benign childhoods, the rule of thumb to avoid becoming an alky is simple, says the evidence: follow Mother Nature, and go with your body's natural daily cycles of alcohol detoxification, i.e:
- Don't drink in the morning
- If you must drink at lunch time, have some lunch too
- Drink with an evening meal

131

Q. Is Dry January a good idea?

A. Well, it depends what you're looking for. If you want to virtue signal, convince yourself that you're not addicted to booze, or wear a hair shirt…then yes, it's a good idea. On the other hand, going without drink doesn't appear to benefit health in the same way as going without food - as in intermittent fasting.

Half a century of medical evidence is clear: wine drinking is exceptionally health-promoting, provided the drinking is moderate and regular. Here's what a review said in 2011:

> There is ample evidence supporting the health benefits associated with regular and moderate consumption of wine, particularly polyphenol-rich red wine. The practice has been associated with a decreased risk of cardiovascular conditions, type 2 diabetes, and many types of cancer.[330]

By 2018, nothing had changed one iota. In a review entitled "Contribution of red wine consumption to human health protection", a team of Czech scientists surveyed 50 years of international data, and voiced a clear message:

> A moderate consumption of wine is recommended daily, mainly with food - about 15 and 30 grams of alcohol for women and men respectively. The highest tolerated dose ranges up to 36 grams per day for healthy women and up to 60 grams per day for healthy men.[331]

So if you, as a daily moderate wine-drinker, "do Dry January" (or any of its month-long clones), it follows you will lose out on a month's worth of "health protection".

On the other hand, you could at least partially redress the balance by ingesting other sources of polyphenols. Two excellent polyphenol-rich foods are olive oil and sugar-free dark chocolate. The problem is that, although these can deliver some of wine's health benefits, they lack wine's special advantages: for example. chocolate won't give you wine's cancer prevention qualities[332], and olive oil won't give you an extra healthy microbiome.[333]

So is Dry January a good idea? Personally. as a moderate wine drinker, I don't think so. But it's your body, your choice.

16

Afterword

Congratulations on getting to the end of this book. I'm aware it's been a bit of a slog through a mountain of research studies, but I make no apologies for subjecting you to the task. The book's subtitle declared its contents to be "authoritative" and I have tried to live up to that claim. All the research data I have cited come from scientists who have published their findings in respectable journals. Although I have tended to highlight studies that contradict the official anti-alcohol narrative, I've been up front about the overall evidence. I've also not ducked those studies which aren't "good news" - for example, cancers of the mouth, throat and gullet, whose risk factors came as a real surprise to me. Also unexpected were the poor results on the benefits of biodynamic viticulture, which I had imagined would be overwhelmingly positive, given the number of vineyards adopting it.

So the book is as authoritative as I have been able to make it, after many deep dives into the published evidence. Much of it challenges the negative stories which seem increasingly to appear in the media. These may have the trappings of science, but, as Chapter 14 demonstrated, they sometimes can be corrupted by ideology.

The ideology being to demonise drinking - by fair means or foul…often foul.

Year by year, country after country, politicised medical authorities have waged ever more draconian campaigns against drinkers, largely based on alcohol's supposed ever-increasing harms to health.

My last book *The Good News About Booze* was a response to my chance discovery that alcohol doesn't put on weight, leading me down the rabbit holes of further health benefits, most of which were unknown to the general public…and none more so than in regard to wine drinking. And latterly, the good news evidence on wine keeps on coming. Hence the need for this present book, which is a serious challenge to the scientific rationality of the current official 'guidelines'.

I strongly suspect that these guidelines are being made more restrictive in order to pave the way for a full-scale war on alcohol, using the tobacco playbook as the model. First alcohol taxes will be hiked, then advertising banned, and finally perhaps pubs and bars remodelled into a kind of drinkers' apartheid. One can imagine legislation requiring licensed premises to provide two segregated areas: a warm, bright, well-furnished one offering alcohol-free drinks, and the other an outdoor windswept lean-to serving booze. In that context, I note that some anti-alcohol activists have claimed that simply being in the mere presence of drinkers is the equivalent of enduring passive smoking.

Indeed, we seem to be already half-way there. No less a body than the World Health Organisation now "recommends" the following:

- Making alcohol less affordable (e.g. by increasing excise taxes)
- Banning or restricting alcohol marketing across all media
- Reducing alcohol availability (e.g. by regulating sale hours)
- Placing health warnings on the labels of alcoholic beverages[334]

Admittedly, this is not the worst example of the WHO's attempts to usurp national sovereignty, but it's an indication of the way officialdom's wind is blowing - straight out of the tobacco playbook.

However, while demonising and *de facto* banning tobacco may be justified on health grounds (although, if people are prepared to harm their health in return for puffing at a stress-reducing substance, that should be their call - again, 'my body, my choice'), the case of alcohol is completely different.

Whereas smokers succumb to dread diseases of which lung cancer is only one, wine drinkers do the reverse. This book has highlighted the main health benefits in cancer, heart disease, diabetes and dementia - crippling and costly diseases which are often prevented by wine drinking.

Anti-alcohol activists try to claim that these benefits are imaginary, largely based on social class. They argue that wine drinkers are more intelligent than the average Joe, and thus are wealthier and more able to take more care of their health, thus skewing the evidence. This is doubtless true, but such claims ignore the results of clinical trials on human experimental subjects, which consistently show beneficial changes on the biomarkers of disease after drinking wine, and indeed other alcoholic drinks too. These laboratory tests of people's blood and urine are objective measures of improved health - unequivocal biological findings from Randomised Controlled or Crossover Trials, the very pinnacles of scientific evidence. Social class is therefore completely irrelevant.

Experiments on animals also provide the same objective evidence: for example, in the case of Alzheimer's disease, wine-drinking rats exhibit significant reductions in beta-amyloid plaques, biomarkers of the disease in the brain.

What's also very clear from the published evidence is that, to alleviate most of alcohol's harms, there is a simple remedy: the B vitamin folate. It's been known for decades that one of alcohol's downsides is to deplete the body of folate, by blocking its release from liver cells,[335] thus making the body potentially vulnerable to cancer, for example.[336] This is not all bad news, however: it means that the adverse consequences of excessive drinking may simply be due to an easily correctable vitamin deficiency. Nevertheless, the fact that the medical authorities breathe not a word of folate's importance as a preventive 'nutraceutical' shows they have no real concern for our health. If they did, they would advise us on the benefits of a judicious intake of wine, coupled with nutritional advice if we over-indulge.

After all, doctors encourage people who over-indulge in junk foods to dose themselves with statins [337] (despite relatively poor evidence of benefit), so why can't they do the same for people who over-indulge in alcohol, by recommending folate supplements?

But, as the recent Covid debacle illustrates, our medical masters' public health policies are not always rationally based.[338]

For example, it's clear that none of the international drinking guidelines mentioned in Chapter 14 are based on science. If they were, for one thing, they would all agree with each other. Were they "plucked out of the air", as one progenitor of the first British guidelines confessed?[339] Or were they decided upon according to the PR clout of a particular country's anti-alcohol pressure groups? Or perhaps to assuage the guilt of a reformed alcoholic who had somehow become a country's Minister of Health one year?

If governments really must issue advice on drinking habits, they should 'follow the science'. As already mentioned, the strongest scientific evidence comes from clinical trials on humans. As a baseline therefore, governments should use the amounts doled out in those trials, many of which have been cited throughout this book. These generally have used a third of a bottle of wine and 3 measures of spirits per day - figures which ironically exceed many countries' current guidelines.

But also note: these may be the minimum amounts needed to produce beneficial biochemical changes in the body.

So, if medical authorities really had our health in mind when giving advice on drinking, they should stipulate these figures as minimum intakes. This of course stands the current guidelines on their head, whose motive is entirely prohibitionist. In a nutshell, their message is "We would prefer you not to drink, but if you really must, don't drink more than ....". It should, of course, be the reverse.

Sadly, as the history of modern public health measures amply testify, medical authorities have a tendency to part company with evidence-based behaviour - for example, continuing to promote low-fat foods despite the diets causing obesity.[340] So it's unlikely that they would do such a dramatic volte-face as to recommend wine drinking, after years of semi-prohibitionist propaganda.

But here's a suggestion. Why don't national governments ignore the medics and follow the science? They don't need to shout the pro-wine message from the rooftops, but they could subtly achieve the same end by one simple measure: taxation. After all, the French already tax wine at minuscule levels (admittedly, mainly to protect an important national industry) but, whatever the motive, the principle of using low taxation to encourage wine-drinking has a strong precedent.

In a rational world therefore, wine should be classified as a food, and thus with zero tax added to its purchase price. To compensate governments for a slight dent in revenue (a tiny fraction of the £10bn from all alcoholic drinks per year in the UK*, and roughly the same in the USA), taxes could be marginally increased on other less healthy alcohols such as spirits. The downside, of course, is that this could lead to an explosion of alcoholism among wine drinkers. That's indeed possible, but unlikely: have you ever known an alcoholic who was an exclusive wine drinker? Frankly, I doubt that such a creature exists.

By contrast, tacitly encouraging wine drinking by eliminating taxes would have enormous health benefits among the wider population, dramatically reducing the incidence of heart disease, diabetes, dementia and even some cancers. On cost grounds alone, the savings to national health expenditures could be substantial - not to mention ending up with a happier and healthier populace.

---

* The UK's £10 billion alcohol tax revenues are more than double the direct costs of dealing with alcohol abuse (e.g. NHS, police and welfare), which amount to less than £4 billion per year. *Source: Institute of Economic Affairs,* 15 Feb 2017

Furthermore, how about governments ditching the drinking guidelines altogether? These are clearly not evidence-based, and guaranteed to impair wine drinkers' health if anyone were foolish enough to follow them.

But of course, it's fanciful to imagine that the authorities would ever do anything so rational. Until there is a revolution in mindless medical demonising. we will doubtless continue to be the recipients of pig-ignorant prohibitionist propaganda.

So when you next read a press story claiming that some supposedly scientific study has found that downing a molecule of alcohol will send you to an early grave, remember that there is an obverse to the old adage that something can sound too good to be true… sounding too bad to be true.

References

1   Bagnardi V et al (2015). Alcohol consumption and site-specific cancer risk: a comprehensive dose–response meta-analysis. *British journal of cancer* 112(3), 580-593.

2   Clinton SK, Giovannucci EL & Hursting SD (2020). The world cancer research fund/American institute for cancer research third expert report on diet, nutrition, physical activity, and cancer: impact and future directions. *The Journal of nutrition,* 150(4), 663-671.

3   WCRF/ AIRC *Continuous Update Project.*

4   Hashibe M et al (2009) Interaction between tobacco and alcohol use and the risk of head and neck cancer: pooled analysis in the International Head and Neck Cancer Epidemiology Consortium. *Cancer Epidemiology and Prevention Biomarkers* 18.2 : 541-550.

5   Stornetta A, Guidolin V & Balbo S (2018) Alcohol-derived acetaldehyde exposure in the oral cavity. *Cancers*, 10(1), 20

6   Gammon MD et al (1997) Tobacco, alcohol, and socioeconomic status and adenocarcinomas of the esophagus and gastric cardia. *J.Natl Cancer Inst.* 3;89(17):1277-84.

7   Barra S et al (1990) Type of alcoholic beverage and cancer of the oral cavity, pharynx and oesophagus in an Italian area with high wine consumption. *International journal of cancer* 46.6 : 1017-1020

8   Bosetti C et al (2000) Wine and other types of alcoholic beverages and the risk of esophageal cancer. *Eur J Clin Nutr* 54, 918–920

9   Kawakita D & Matsuo K (2017) Alcohol and head and neck cancer. *Cancer and Metastasis Reviews*, 36, 425-434.

10   Purdue MP et al (2009) Type of alcoholic beverage and risk of head and neck cancer—a pooled analysis within the INHANCE Consortium.*American Journal of Epidemiology*, *169*(2), 132-142.

11   Kubo A et al (2009) Alcohol types and sociodemographic characteristics as risk factors for Barrett's esophagus *Gastroenterology.* 136(3): 806–815

12   Thrift AP et al (2011) Lifetime alcohol consumption and risk of Barrett's Esophagus. *American Journal of Gastroenterology*, 106(7), 1220-1230.

13   Yang Q et al (2009) Serum folate and cancer mortality among US adults: findings from the Third National Health and Nutritional Examination Survey linked mortality file. *Cancer Epidemiology and Prevention Biomarkers,* 18(5), 1439-1447

14   Larsson S et al (2006) Folate intake, MTHFR polymorphisms, and risk of esophageal, gastric, and pancreatic cancer: a meta-analysis. *Gastroenterology* 131.4 : 1271-1283

15   Liu W, Zhou H, Zhu Y, Tie C (2017) Associations between dietary folate intake and risks of esophageal, gastric and pancreatic cancers: an overall and dose-response meta-analysis. *Oncotarget.* Jun 28;8(49):86828-86842.

16   Galeone C et al (2006) Folate intake and squamous-cell carcinoma of the oesophagus in Italian and Swiss men. *Annals of Oncology,* 17(3), 521-525.

17   Matsuo K et al (2012) Folate, alcohol, and aldehyde dehydrogenase 2 polymorphism and the risk of oral and pharyngeal cancer in Japanese. *European Journal of Cancer Prevention*, 21(2), 193-198

18   Hwang PH et al (2012) Alcohol intake and folate antagonism via CYP2E1 and ALDH1: Effects on oral carcinogenesis. *Medical Hypotheses,* 78(2), 197-202.

19   Turati F et al (2014) Alcohol and liver cancer: a systematic review and meta-analysis of prospective studies *Annals of Oncology* 25: 1526-1535

20   Turati F et al (2014) op cit

21   Lieber CS (1991) Hepatic, Metabolic and Toxic Effects of Ethanol: Update *Alcoholism: Clinical and Experimental Research* 15 (4) 573–92

22   Rehm J et al (2010). Alcohol as a risk factor for liver cirrhosis - a systematic review and meta-analysis. *Drug Alcohol Rev.* ;29:437–445

23   Blachier M et al (2013) The burden of liver disease in Europe: a review of available epidemiological data. *Journal of Hepatology* 58.3: 593-608

24   Becker U et al (1996) Prediction of risk of liver disease by alcohol intake, sex and age: a prospective population study. *Hepatology* 23:1025–1029

25   Sørensen TI et al (1984) Prospective evaluation of alcohol abuse and alcoholic liver injury in men as predictors of development of cirrhosis *Lancet* 4;2(8397):241-4

26   Stokkeland K et al (2008) Different drinking patterns for women and men with alcohol dependence with and without alcoholic cirrhosis *Alcohol Alcohol* ;43:39-45

27   Mann RE et al (2003) The epidemiology of alcoholic liver disease. *Alcohol research & health,* 27(3), 209.

28   Dawson DA (2000). Drinking patterns among individuals with and without DSM-IV alcohol use disorders. *Journal of Studies on Alcohol,* 61(1), 111-120.

29   Grønbæk M et al (2004) Intake of beer, wine and spirits and risk of heavy drinking and alcoholic cirrhosis. *Biological Research,* 37(2), 195-200

30   Bellentani S et al (1997) Drinking habits as cofactors of risk for alcohol induced liver damage. *Gut,* 41(6), 845-850.

31   Monzoni A et al (2001) Genetic determinants of ethanol-induced liver damage *Mol Med.* 7(4):255-62.

32   Seitz HK et al (2018) Alcoholic liver disease. *Nature reviews Disease primers,* 4(1), 16.

33   McNabb S et al (2020) Meta-analysis of 16 studies of the association of alcohol with colorectal cancer. *International journal of cancer,* 146(3), 861-873

34   Vecchia CL et al (1993) Refined-sugar intake and the risk of colorectal cancer in humans. *International Journal of Cancer* 55.3 : 386-389

35   Crockett SD et al (2011) Inverse relationship between moderate alcohol intake and rectal cancer: analysis of the North Carolina Colon Cancer Study. *Diseases of the Colon and Rectum,* 54(7), 887.

36   Park JY et al (2009) Baseline alcohol consumption, type of alcoholic beverage and risk of colorectal cancer in the European

Prospective Investigation into Cancer and Nutrition-Norfolk study. *Cancer Epidemiology*, 33(5), 347-354

37   Queipo-Ortuno M et al (2012) Influence of red wine polyphenols and ethanol on gut microbiota ecology and biochemical biomarkers. *Am J Clin Nutr* 95(6):1323-34

38   Xu W et al. (2019). Wine consumption and colorectal cancer risk: a meta-analysis of observational studies. *European Journal of Cancer Prevention*, 28(3), 151-158.

39   SEER Cancer Statistics Review,1975-2013 (2016) *National Cancer Institute*.

40   Schoonen WM et al (2005) Alcohol consumption and risk of prostate cancer in middle-aged men. *International Journal of Cancer* 113(1), 133-140

41   Vartolomei MH et al (2018) The impact of moderate wine consumption on the risk of developing prostate cancer. *Clinical Epidemiology* 10: 431-44

42   Downer MK et al (2019). Alcohol intake and risk of lethal prostate cancer in the Health Professionals Follow-Up Study. *Journal of Clinical Oncology,* 37(17), 1499-1511.

43   Kampa M et al (2000). Wine antioxidant polyphenols inhibit the proliferation of human prostate cancer cell lines. *Nutrition and cancer,* 37(2), 223-33

44   Brizuel L et al (2010) esphingosine kinase-1 survival pathway is a molecular target for the tumor-suppressive tea and wine polyphenols in prostate cancer. *FASEB Journal,* 24(10), 3882-94

45   Chao C et al (2008) Alcoholic beverage intake and risk of lung cancer: the California Men's Health Study. *Cancer Epidemiology Biomarkers & Prevention,* 17(10), 2692-2699.

46   Brenner DR et al (2019) Alcohol consumption and lung cancer risk: A pooled analysis from the International Lung Cancer Consortium and the SYNERGY study. *Cancer epidemiology,* 58, 25-32.

47   Schwarz V et al (2017) Red Wine Prevents the Acute Negative Vascular Effects of Smoking. *American Journal of Medicine* 130.1: 95-100

48   Barstad B et al (2005) Intake of Wine, Beer and Spirits and Risk of Gastric Cancer *Eur J Cancer Prev* ; 14(3):239-43.

49   Wang, PL et al (2017) Alcohol drinking and gastric cancer risk: a meta-analysis of observational studies. *Oncotarget* 8.58: 99013

50   Wang Y-T et al (2016) Association between alcohol intake and the risk of pancreatic cancer: a dose–response meta-analysis of cohort studies. *BMC cancer* 16.1: 212.

51   Herreros-Villanueva M et al (2013) Alcohol consumption on pancreatic diseases. *World J Gastroenterol* 19(5):638–647

52   Larsson SC (2006) op cit.

53   ACS website, accessed August 2023.

54   WHO website accessed August 2023

55   Ingold N, Amin H A, Drenos F (2019) Alcohol causes an increased risk of head and neck but not breast cancer in individuals from the UK Biobank study: A Mendelian randomisation analysis. *medRxiv*, 19002832

56   Bessaoud F & Daures JP (2008) Patterns of alcohol (especially wine) consumption and breast cancer risk: a case-control study among a population in Southern France. *Annals of Epidemiology,* 18(6), 467-475.

57   Mourouti N et al (2014) The J-shaped Association Between Alcohol Consumption and Breast in Cancer: A Case-Control Study *Current Nutrition & Food Science* Volume 10, Issue 2; 120 - 127

58   Newcomb PA et al (2009) No difference between red wine or white wine consumption and breast cancer risk. *Cancer Epidemiology Biomarkers & Prevention,* 18(3), 1007-1010

59   Shufelt C et al (2012) Red versus white wine as a nutritional aromatase inhibitor in premenopausal women: a pilot study. *Journal of women's health,* 21(3), 281-284.

60   Weng ET et al (2002) Anti-Aromatase Chemicals in Red Wine. *Annals of the New York Academy of Sciences,* 963(1), 239-246.

61   Boyd NF et al (1998) Mammographic densities and breast cancer risk. *Cancer Epidemiology Biomarkers & Prevention, (*712), 1133-1144.

62   Flom JD et al (2009) Alcohol intake over the life course and mammographic density. *Breast cancer research and treatment,* 117(3), 643-651.

63   Chen J-Y et al (2016) Dose-Dependent Associations between Wine Drinking and Breast Cancer Risk-Meta-Analysis Findings. *Asian Pac J Cancer Prev* 17.3: 1221-1233.

64   Hill AB (1965) The environment and disease: association or causation? *Proc R Soc Med.* 58:295–300.

65   Boccia S et al (2009) Aldehyde dehydrogenase 2 and head and neck cancer: a meta-analysis implementing a Mendelian randomization approach. *Cancer Epidemiology Biomarkers & Prevention,* 18(1), 248-254.

66   Borja-Oliveira C (2014) Alcohol-medication interactions: the acetaldehyde syndrome. *J Pharmacovigilance, 2*(145), 2.

67   Fraser GE et al (2020) Dairy, soy, and risk of breast cancer: those confounded milks. *International Journal of Epidemiology* 49.5 : 1526-1537.

68   Kakkoura MG et al (2022) Dairy consumption and risks of total and site-specific cancers in Chinese adults: an 11-year prospective study of 0.5 million people. *BMC medicine,* 20(1), 1-13.

69   Kim HJ et al (2017) Alcohol consumption and breast cancer risk in younger women according to family history of breast cancer and folate intake. *American Journal of Epidemiology* 186.5 (2017): 524-531.

70   Sellers TA et al (2001) Dietary folate intake, alcohol, and risk of breast cancer in a prospective study of postmenopausal women. *Epidemiology,* 420-428

71   Gómez-Revuelta C (2018) Alcohol and folate intake association with breast cancer: a metanalysis. *UCREA Académico*

72   Stolzenberg-Solomon RZ et al (2006) Folate intake, alcohol use, and postmenopausal breast cancer risk in the Prostate, Lung, Colorectal, and Ovarian Cancer Screening Trial. *The American Journal of Clinical Nutrition,* 83(4), 895-904.

73   Pelucchi C et al (2008) Alcohol consumption and renal cell cancer risk in two Italian case-control studies *Ann Oncol.* 19(5):1003-8.

74   Yuan H C et al (2021). Alcohol intake and the risk of chronic kidney disease: results from a systematic review and dose–response meta-analysis. European Journal of Clinical Nutrition, 75(11), 1555-1567.

75   Hu EA et al (2020)Alcohol consumption and incident kidney disease: results from the atherosclerosis risk in communities study. *Journal of Renal Nutrition* 30.1 : 22-30

76   Burchfiel CM et al (1997) Cardiovascular risk factors and hyalinization of renal arterioles at autopsy   *Arteriosclerosis, thrombosis, and vascular biology* 17.4: 760-768.

77   Meinhold CL (2009) Alcohol intake and risk of thyroid cancer in the NIH-AARP Diet and Health Study *Br J Cancer.* 3;101(9):1630-4

78   Hong SH et al (2017) Alcohol intake and risk of thyroid cancer: a meta-analysis of observational studies. *Cancer research and treatment: official journal of Korean Cancer Association,* 49(2), 534.

79   Chiu BC et al (1999) Alcohol consumption and non-Hodgkin lymphoma in a cohort of older women.*Br J Cancer.* 80(9): 1476–1482.

80   Morton LM et al (2005) Alcohol consumption and risk of non-Hodgkin lymphoma: a pooled analysis. *Lancet Oncol.* 6(7):469-76

81   Gapstur SM et al (2012) Alcohol intake and the incidence of Non-Hodgkin lymphoid neoplasms in the cancer prevention study II nutrition cohort *Am J Epidemiol.* 176(1):60-9

82   Sundquist J & Sundquist K (2014) Alcohol consumption has a protective effect against hematological malignancies: a population based study in Sweden including 420,489 individuals with alcohol use disorders.*Neoplasia.* Mar; 16(3): 229–234

83   Andreotti G et al (2013) A pooled analysis of alcohol consumption and risk of multiple myeloma in the international multiple myeloma consortium *Cancer Epidemiol Biomarkers Prev*; 22(9); 1620–7

84   Psaltopoulou T et al (2015) Alcohol intake, alcoholic beverage type and multiple myeloma risk: a meta-analysis of 26 observational studies. *Leukemia & Lymphoma,* 56(5), 1484-1501.

85   Renaud SD & De Lorgeril M (1992). Wine, alcohol, platelets, and the French paradox for coronary heart disease. *Lancet*, 339(8808), 1523-26.

86   Doll R et al (1994) Mortality in relation to consumption of alcohol: 13 years' observations on male British doctors. *British Medical Journal*, 309(6959), 911-8.

87   Abramson JL et al (2001) Moderate alcohol consumption and risk of heart failure among older persons. *JAMA*, 285(15), 1971-77

88   Gillman MW et al (1995) Relationship of alcohol intake with blood pressure in young adults. *Hypertension*, 25(5), 1106-1110

89   Sacco RL et al (1999) The protective effect of moderate alcohol consumption on ischemic stroke. *JAMA*, 281(1), 53-60.

90   Hackney AC, Koltun KJ (2012) The immune system and overtraining in athletes: clinical implications. *Acta clinica Croatica*, 51(4.), 633-640.

91   Lian C (1915) L'alcoolisme, cause d'hypertension arterielle. *Bull Acad Med* 74: 525-28

92   Patra J et al (2010) Alcohol consumption and the risk of morbidity and mortality for different stroke types - a systematic review and meta-analysis *BMC Public Health* 10:258

93   Ibid.

94   Kodama S et al (2011) Alcohol consumption and risk of atrial fibrillation. A meta-analysis. *J Am Coll Cardiol* 57:427–436

95   Kiechl S et al (1998) Alcohol consumption and atherosclerosis: what is the relation? *Stroke* 29.5: 900-907

96   Piano MR (2002) Alcoholic cardiomyopathy: incidence, clinical characteristics and pathophysiology *Chest* 121:1638–1650

97   Shaper AG, Wannamethee G, Walker M (1988) Alcohol and mortality in British men: explaining the U-shaped curve. *Lancet*, 332(8623), 1267-1273

98   Fillmore KM et al (2007) Moderate alcohol use and reduced mortality risk: systematic error in prospective studies and new hypotheses. *Annals of epidemiology*, 17(5), S16-S23.

99   Rimm EB et al (1991) Prospective study of alcohol consumption and risk of coronary disease in men. *Lancet.* 338(8765):464-8.

100   Mukamal KJ, Chiuve SE, Rimm EB (2006) Alcohol consumption and risk for coronary heart disease in men with healthy lifestyles. *Archives of Internal Medicine*, 166(19), 2145-50.

101   Rimm EB et al (1999) Moderate alcohol intake and lower risk of coronary heart disease: metaanalysis of effects on lipids and haemostatic factors. *BMJ* 319(7224),1523.

102   Ronksley PE et al (2011) Association of alcohol consumption with selected cardiovascular disease outcomes: a systematic review and meta analysis. *BMJ*: 342, d671

103   Fuller TD (2011) Moderate alcohol consumption and the risk of mortality. *Demography.* 48(3):1105-25

104   Roerecke M, Rehm J (2012) The cardioprotective association of average alcohol consumption and ischaemic heart disease: a systematic review and meta-analysis *Addiction* 107.7: 1246-1260.

105   Rimm EB, Moats C (2007) Alcohol and Coronary Heart Disease: Drinking Patterns and Mediators of Effect *Ann Epidemiol*;17:S3–S7

106   Boffetta P, Garfinkel L (1990) Alcohol drinking and mortality among men enrolled in an American Cancer Society prospective study. *Epidemiology* 1.5 342-348

107   Klatsky AL, Armstrong M, Friedman GD (1990) Risk of cardiovascular mortality in alcohol drinkers, ex-drinkers and nondrinkers. *Am J Cardiol;*66:1237-1242.

108   Stampfer MJ et al (1998) Prospective study of moderate alcohol consumption and the risk of coronary disease and stroke in women. *N Engl J Med.* 319:267-273.

109   Boffetta P, Garfinkel L (1990) Alcohol drinking and mortality among men enrolled in an American Cancer Society prospective study. *Epidemiology.* 1:342-348

110   Rimm EB et al (1991) Prospective study of alcohol consumption and risk of coronary heart disease in men. *Lancet* 338:464-468.

111   Klatsky AL, Armstrong MA, Friedman GD (1992) Alcohol and mortality. *Ann Intern Med.*117:646-654.

112   Blackwelder WC et al (1980) Alcohol and mortality: the Honolulu Heart study. *Am J Med.;*68:164-169

113   Jackson R, Scragg R, Beaglehole R (1991) Alcohol consumption and risk of coronary heart disease. *BMJ.* 303:211-216.

114   Kiechl S et al (1998) Alcohol consumption and atherosclerosis: what is the relation? Prospective results from the Bruneck Study. *Stroke*, 29(5), 900-907.

115   Merchant AT et al (2008) Interrelation of saturated fat, trans fat, alcohol intake, and subclinical atherosclerosis. *The American journal of clinical nutrition*, 87(1), 168-74

116   Brunner FJ et al (2019) Application of non-HDL cholesterol for population-based cardiovascular risk stratification: results from the Multinational Cardiovascular Risk Consortium. *The Lancet,* 394 (10215), 2173-83.

117   Brien SE et al (2011) Effect of alcohol consumption on biological markers associated with risk of coronary heart disease: systematic review and meta-analysis of interventional studies. *BMJ*, 342, d636

118   Mukamal KJ et al (2005) Alcohol consumption and platelet activation and aggregation among women and men: the Framingham Offspring Study. *Alcoholism: Clinical and Experimental Research,* 29(10), 1906-1912.

119   Walker RK et al (2013) The good, the bad and the ugly with alcohol use and abuse on the heart. *Alcohol Clin Exp Res.* (8): 1253–1260.

120   Bau PF et al (2007) Alcohol consumption, cardiovascular health, and endothelial function markers. *Alcohol*, 41(7), 479-488

121   Rimm EB, Moats C. (2007) Alcohol and coronary heart disease: drinking patterns and mediators of effect. *Annals of Epidemiology*, 17(5), S3-S7.

122   Van de Luitgaarden IA et al (2021) Alcohol consumption in relation to cardiovascular diseases and mortality: a systematic review of Mendelian randomization studies. *European journal of epidemiology*, 1-15

123   Mukamal KJ, Stampfer MJ & Rimm EB (2020) Genetic instrumental variable analysis: time to call Mendelian Randomization what it is. *Eur J Epidemiol* 35, 93–97

124   Rimm EB, Klatsky A, Grobbee D, Stampfer MJ (1996). Review of moderate alcohol consumption and reduced risk of coronary heart disease: is the effect due to beer, wine, or liquor?. *BMJ*, 312(7033), 731-736.

125   Estruch R et al (2004). Different effects of red wine and gin consumption on inflammatory biomarkers of atherosclerosis: a prospective randomized crossover trial: effects of wine on inflammatory markers. *Atherosclerosis*, 175(1), 117-123.

126   Chiva-Blanch G et al (2012) Effects of red wine polyphenols and alcohol on glucose metabolism and the lipid profile: a randomized clinical trial. *Clinical Nutrition*, 32(2), 200-206.

127   Estruch R et al (2011) Moderate consumption of red wine, but not gin, decreases erythrocyte superoxide dismutase activity: a randomised cross-over trial. *Nutrition, Metabolism and Cardiovascular Diseases*, 21(1), 46-53.

128   Badia E et al (2010) Decreased tumor necrosis factor-induced adhesion of human monocytes to endothelial cells after moderate alcohol consumption *Cell Physiol Biochem.* 26(3):471-82

129   Sacanella E et al (2007) Down-regulation of adhesion molecules and other inflammatory biomarkers after moderate wine consumption in healthy women: a randomized trial. *The American journal of clinical nutrition*, 86(5), 1463-1469.

130   Roerecke M, Rehm J (2014). Alcohol consumption, drinking patterns, and ischemic heart disease: a narrative review of meta-analyses *BMC medicine* 12.1: 182.

131   Le Strat Y, Gorwood P (2011) Hazardous drinking is associated with a lower risk of coronary heart disease: results from a national representative sample *Am J Addict.* 20(3):257-63

132   Arriola L et al (2010) Alcohol intake and the risk of coronary heart disease in the Spanish EPIC cohort study *Heart.* 96(2):124-30.

133   Renaud SC et al (2004) Moderate wine drinkers have lower hypertension-related mortality: a prospective cohort study in French men. *The American journal of clinical nutrition*, 80(3), 621-625.

134   Rifler JP et al (2012) A moderate red wine intake improves blood lipid parameters and erythrocytes membrane fluidity in post myocardial infarct patients. *Molecular nutrition & food research*, 56(2), 345-351

135   Dixon JB, Dixon ME & O'Brien PE (2002) Reduced plasma homocysteine in obese red wine consumers: a potential contributor to reduced cardiovascular risk status. *European journal of clinical nutrition*, 56(7), 608-614.

136   Di Giuseppe R et al (2009) Alcohol consumption and n–3 polyunsaturated fatty acids in healthy men and women from 3 European populations *Am J Clin Nutr*; 89:354–62.

137   Harris WS et al (2017) The Omega-3 Index and relative risk for coronary heart disease mortality: Estimation from 10 cohort studies. *Atherosclerosis*, 262, 51-54.

138   Li XH et al (2016) Association between alcohol consumption and the risk of incident type 2 diabetes: a systematic review and dose-response meta-analysis. *The American journal of clinical nutrition*, 103(3), 818-829.

139   Pietraszek A, Gregersen S, Hermansen K (2010) Alcohol and type 2 diabetes. A review. *Nutr Metab Cardiovasc Dis.* ;20(5):366-75

140   Huang J, Wang X & Zhang Y (2017) Specific types of alcoholic beverage consumption and risk of type 2 diabetes: A systematic review and meta-analysis. *Journal of diabetes investigation*, 8(1), 56-68.

141   Avogaro A, Tiengo A (1993) Alcohol, glucose metabolism and diabetes. *Diabetes/metabolism reviews*, 9(2), 129-146.

142   Kiechl S et al (1996) Insulin sensitivity and regular alcohol consumption: large prospective, cross-sectional population study *BMJ*, 313, 1040-1044

143   Carlsson S, Hammar N & Grill V (2005) Alcohol consumption and type 2 diabetes. *Diabetologia* 48, 1051–1054

144   Sierksma A et al (2004) Effect of moderate alcohol consumption on adiponectin, tumor necrosis factor-⟨, and insulin sensitivity. *Diabetes Care*, 27(1), 184-189.

145   Zelle DM et al (2011) Alcohol consumption, new onset of diabetes after transplantation, and all-cause mortality in renal transplant recipients *Transplantation.* 27;92(2):203-9.

146   Blomster JI et al (2014) The relationship between alcohol consumption and vascular complications and mortality in individuals with type 2 diabetes. *Diabetes care*, 37(5), 1353-1359.

147   Napoli R et al (2005) Red wine consumption improves insulin resistance but not endothelial function in type 2 diabetic patients. *Metabolism*, 54(3), 306-313.

148   Mozumdar A, Liguori G (2011) Persistent increase of prevalence of metabolic syndrome among US adults: NHANES III to NHANES 1999–2006. *Diabetes care* 34.1: 216-219.

149   Alkerwi A et al (2009) Alcohol consumption and the prevalence of metabolic syndrome: a meta-analysis of observational studies. *Atherosclerosis* 204.2 (2009): 624-635.

150   Gepner Y et al (2015) Effects of initiating moderate alcohol intake on cardiometabolic risk in adults with type 2 diabetes: a 2-year randomized, controlled trial. *Annals of internal medicine*, 163(8), 569-579.

151   Mehlig K et al (2008) Alcoholic beverages and incidence of dementia: 34-year follow-up of the prospective population study of women in Göteborg. *American journal of epidemiology*, 167(6), 684-691.

152   Truelsen T, Thudium D & Grønbæk M (2002) Amount and type of alcohol and risk of dementia The Copenhagen City Heart Study. *Neurology*, 59(9), 1313-1319.

153   Letenneur L (2004) Risk of dementia and alcohol and wine consumption: a review of recent results. *Biological research*, 37(2), 189-194.

154   Pasinetti GM (2012) Novel role of red wine-derived polyphenols in the prevention of Alzheimer's disease, dementia and brain pathology: experimental approaches and clinical implications. *Planta medica,* 1614-1619

155   Gu Y et al (2014) Alcohol intake and brain structure in a multiethnic elderly cohort. *Clin Nutr* 33(4):662-7

156   Zuccala G et al (2001) Dose-related impact of alcohol consumption on cognitive function in advanced age: results of a multicenter survey *Alcohol Clin Exp Res;* 25:1743–1748.

157   Schaefer SM et al (2022). Association of alcohol types, coffee, and tea intake with risk of dementia: prospective cohort study of UK Biobank participants *Brain Sciences*, 12(3), 360.

158   Baraona E et al (2001) Gender differences in pharmacokinetics of alcohol. *Alcoholism: Clinical and Experimental Research*, 25(4), 502-507.

159   Frezza M et al. (1990) High blood alcohol levels in women: the role of decreased gastric alcohol dehydrogenase

activity and first-pass metabolism. *New England Journal of Medicine,* 322(2), 95-99

160   Chrostek L et al. (2003). Gender-related differences in hepatic activity of alcohol dehydrogenase isoenzymes and aldehyde dehydrogenase in humans. *Journal of clinical laboratory analysis,* 17(3), 93-96.

161   Agarwal D P, Harada S, & Goedde H W. (1981). Racial differences in biological sensitivity to ethanol: the role of alcohol dehydrogenase and aldehyde dehydrogenase isozymes. *Alcoholism: Clinical and Experimental Research,* 5(1), 12-16.

162   Agarwal D P et al (1984). Basis of aldehyde dehydrogenase deficiency in Orientals: immunochemical studies. *Alcohol,* 1(2), 111-118

163   Peng G S & Yin S J (2009). Effect of the allelic variants of aldehyde dehydrogenase ALDH2* 2 and alcohol dehydrogenase ADH1B* 2 on blood acetaldehyde concentrations. *Human genomics, 3,* 1-7.

164   Neumark YD et al. (2004). Alcohol dehydrogenase polymorphisms influence alcohol-elimination rates in a male Jewish population. *Alcoholism: Clinical and Experimental Research,* 28(1), 10-14.

165   Luo HR et al (2009) Origin and dispersal of atypical aldehyde dehydrogenase *Gene,* 435(1), 96-103

166   Goedde HW, Harada S & Agarwal DP (1979). Racial differences in alcohol sensitivity: a new hypothesis. *Human genetics,* 51, 331-334.

167   USDA & USDHHS Dietary Guidelines for Americans, 2010. 7th Edition, Washington, DC: U.S. Government Printing Office, December 2010.

168   *USA Today* 15 Nov 2015

169   British Nutrition Foundation Press Release, April 2009

170   Smith RR et al (2009) Ethanol consumption does not promote weight gain in female mice. *Annals of Nutrition and Metabolism,* 53(3- 4), 252-259.

171   Aguiar AS, Da-Silva VA & Boaventura GT (2004) Can calories from ethanol contribute to body weight preservation by malnourished rats?. Brazilian journal of medical and biological research, 37, 841-846.

172   Hackney JF, Engelman RM, Good RA (1992) Ethanol calories do not enhance breast cancer in isocalorically fed C3H/Ou mice. *Nutrition & Cancer,* 18(3):245-53

173   Monteiro R et al (2009) Red wine increases adipose tissue aromatase expression and regulates body weight and adipocyte size. *Nutrition*, 25(6), 699-705

174   Cordain L, Bryan ED, Melby CL, Smith MJ (1997) Influence of moderate daily wine consumption on body weight regulation and metabolism in healthy free-living males. *Journal of the American College of Nutrition*, 16(2), 134-139

175   MacInnis RJ et al (2014) Predictors of increased body weight and waist circumference for middle-aged adults. *Public health nutrition*, 17(5), 1087-1097.

176   Tomson CA et al (2012) Alcohol consumption and body weight change in postmenopausal women: results from the Women's Health Initiative.*International Journal of Obesity*, 36(9), 1158-1164.

177   Lieber CS (1991) Perspectives: do alcohol calories count? *American Journal of Clinical Nutrition,* 54(6), 976-82.

178   Taller H (1961) 'Calories Don't Count', Heinemann

179   Brand-Miller JC et al (2002) Glycemic index and obesity. *The American journal of clinical nutrition*, 76(1), 281S-285S.

180   Taubes G (2008) 'The Diet Delusion', Ebury Publishing

181   Harcombe Z (2011) 'The Obesity Epidemic', Columbus Publishing

182   Spector T (2020) 'Spoon-Fed', Jonathan Cape.

183   Ludwig DS (2002) The glycemic index: physiological mechanisms relating to obesity, diabetes, and cardiovascular disease. *JAMA*, 287(18), 2414-2423

184   Guarneiri LL, Cooper JA (2020) Intake of nuts or nut products does not lead to weight gain, independent of dietary substitution instructions: A systematic review and meta-analysis of randomized trials. *Advances in Nutrition* 12(2), 384-401.

185 National Institute on Alcohol Abuse and Alcoholism No. 22 PH 346 October 1993 274 CDC Fact Sheets

186   Valdes AM et al (2018) Role of the gut microbiota in nutrition and health. *BMJ* 361.k2179.

187   Spector T (2020) op. cit.

188   Das B, Nair GB (2019) Homeostasis and dysbiosis of the gut microbiome in health and disease. *Journal of biosciences*, 44(5), 1-8.

189   Barroso E et al (2017) Phylogenetic profile of gut microbiota in healthy adults after moderate intake of red wine, *Mol. Nutr. Food Res.* 61, 1600620

190   Queipo-Ortuño MI et al (2012) Influence of red wine polyphenols and ethanol on the gut microbiota ecology and biochemical biomarkers. *The American journal of clinical nutrition*, 95(6), 1323-1334.

191   Spector T (2020) op. cit.

192   Le Roy CI et al (2020) Red wine consumption associated with increased gut microbiota α-diversity in 3 independent cohorts. *Gastroenterology*, 158(1), 270-272.

193   Del Rio D, Stewart AJ & Pellegrini N (2005) A review of recent studies on malondialdehyde as toxic molecule and biological marker of oxidative stress. *Nutrition, metabolism and cardiovascular diseases,* 15(4), 316-328.

194   Gorelik S et al (2008) The stomach as a "bioreactor": when red meat meets red wine. *Journal of agricultural and food chemistry,* 56(13), 5002-5007.

195   Choi TY et al (2020) Mental disorders linked to crosstalk between the gut microbiome and the brain. *Experimental Neurobiology*, 29(6), 403

196   Moreno-Arribas MV et al (2020) Relationship between wine consumption, diet and microbiome modulation in Alzheimer's disease. *Nutrients*, 12(10), 3082.

197   Filosa S et al (2018) Polyphenols-gut microbiota interplay and brain neuromodulation. *Neural regeneration research*, 13(12), 2055.

198   Spector T (2020) op. cit.

199   Wu CJ et al (2007) Comparison of prevalence between self-reported erectile dysfunction. *Urology*, 69(4), 743-747.

200   Mondaini N et al (2009) Regular moderate intake of red wine is linked to better women's sexual health. *The Journal of Sexual Medicine*, 6(10), 2772-2777.

201   Crispo A et al (2004) Alcohol and the risk of prostate cancer and benign prostatic hyperplasia. *Urology*, 64(4), 717-722.

202   Parsons JK & I R (2009). Alcohol consumption is associated with a decreased risk of benign prostatic hyperplasia. *The Journal of urology*, 182(4), 1463-1468.

203   Diaz-Cruz C et al (2017) The effect of alcohol and red wine consumption on clinical and MRI outcomes in multiple sclerosis. *Multiple sclerosis and related disorders*, 17, 47-53.

204   Muthuri SG et al (2015) Beer and wine consumption and risk of knee or hip osteoarthritis: a case control study. *Arthritis research & therapy*, 17(1), 1-14.

205   Turk JN et al (2021) Exploring the effect of alcohol on disease activity and outcomes in rheumatoid arthritis through systematic review and meta-analysis. *Scientific Reports*, 11(1), 1-6..

206   Cohen S et al (1993) Smoking, alcohol consumption, and susceptibility to the common cold. *American journal of public health*, 83(9), 1277-1283.

207   Takkouche B et al (2002) Intake of wine, beer, and spirits and the risk of clinical common cold. *American Journal of Epidemiology*, 155(9), 853-858.

208   Tucker KL et al (2009) Effects of beer, wine, and liquor intakes on bone mineral density in older men and women. The American journal of clinical nutrition, 89(4), 1188-1196.

209   Ciubara AB et al (2018) The composition of bioactive compounds in wine and their possible influence on osteoporosis and on bone consolidation. *Revista de Chimie,* 69(5), 1247-1253.

210   Misciagna G et al (1996) Epidemiology of cholelithiasis in southern Italy. Part II: Risk factors. *European journal of gastroenterology & hepatology*, 8(6), 585-594.

211   Cha BH et al (2019) Alcohol consumption can reduce the risk of gallstone disease: a systematic review with a dose-response meta-analysis of case-control and cohort studies. *Gut and Liver*, 13(1), 114.

212   Curhan GC et al (1998) Beverage use and risk for kidney stones in women. *Annals of internal medicine*, 128(7), 534-540.

213   Obisesan TO et al (1998) Moderate wine consumption is associated with decreased odds of developing age-related macular

degeneration in NHANES-1. *Journal of the American Geriatrics Society*, *46*(1), 1-7.

214   Sasaki H et al (2005) The Protective Effect of Wine Intake on Five Year's Incidence of Cataract [Reykjavik Eye Study] *Investigative Ophthalmology & Visual Science*, 46(13), 3840-3840.

215   Chua SY et al (2021) Alcohol consumption and incident cataract surgery in two large UK cohorts. *Ophthalmology,* 128(6), 837-847.

216   Muñoz-González I et al (2014) Red Wine and Oenological Extracts Display Antimicrobial Effects in an Oral Bacteria Biofilm Model *J. Agric. Food Chem.* 62, 20, 4731–4737

217   Doll R et al (1994) Mortality in relation to consumption of alcohol: 13 years' observations on male British doctors *BMJ* 309:911-8

218   Grønbæk M et al (1995) Mortality associated with moderate intakes of wine, beer, or spirits. *BMJ*, 310(6988), 1165-1169.

219   Grønbæk M et al (2000). Type of alcohol consumed and mortality from all causes, coronary heart disease, and cancer. *Annals of Internal Medicine*, 133(6), 411-419.

220   La Vecchia C et al (1995) Prevalence of chronic diseases in alcohol abstainers. *Epidemiology.* 6(4):436-8.

221   Farchi G et al (2000) Alcohol and survival in the Italian rural cohorts of the Seven Countries Study *International journal of epidemiology* 29.4: 667-671

222   Ruf JC (2002) Overview of epidemiological studies on wine, health and mortality *Drugs under experimental and clinical research* 29.5-6: 173-179

223   Renaud SC et al (1999) Wine, beer, and mortality in middle-aged men from eastern France. *Arch Intern Med.* 159(16):1865-70

224   Streppel MT et al (2009) Long-term wine consumption is related to cardiovascular mortality and life expectancy independently of moderate alcohol intake: the Zutphen Study. *J Epidemiol Community Health.* 63(7):534-40.

225   Klatsky AL et al (2003) Wine, liquor, beer, and mortality. *American Journal of Epidemiology*, 158(6), 585-595

226   Dinu M et al (2018) Mediterranean diet and multiple health outcomes: an umbrella review of meta-analyses of observational studies and randomised trials. *Eur J Clin Nutr* 72, 30–43

227   Bonaccio M et al (2016) Adherence to the traditional Mediterranean diet and mortality in subjects with diabetes. Prospective results from the MOLI-SANI study. *Eur J Prev Cardiol* 23(4) 400-7

228   Leon-Muñoz LM et al (2017) Alcohol drinking patterns and risk of functional limitations in two cohorts of older adults. *Clinical nutrition* 36.3: 831-83

229   Sun Q et al (2011) Alcohol consumption at midlife and successful ageing in women: a prospective cohort analysis in the nurses' health study. *PLoS Med* 8.9 : e1001090.

230   Byles J et al (2006) A drink to healthy aging: The association between older women's use of alcohol and their health-related quality of life. *J Am Geriatr Soc.* 54(9):1341-7

231   Grønbaek M et al (1998) Alcohol and mortality: is there a U-shaped relation in elderly people? *Age and Ageing* 27.6: 739-744.

232   Streppel M T et al (2009) *op. cit.*

233   Gambini J et al (2021) Moderate red wine consumption increases the expression of longevity-associated genes in controlled human populations and extends lifespan in Drosophila melanogaster. *Antioxidants*, 10(2), 301

234   Davies S quoted in *The Daily Telegraph* 8th Jan 2016.

235   Ma H et al (2021) Alcohol consumption levels as compared with drinking habits in predicting all-cause mortality and cause-specific mortality in current drinkers. *Mayo Clinic Proceedings* 96, (7), 1758-1769.

236   Jani BD et al (2021) Association between patterns of alcohol consumption (beverage type, frequency and consumption with food) and risk of adverse health outcomes: a prospective cohort study. *BMC medicine*, 19(1), 1-14

237   Schaefer S et al (2023) Association of alcohol types, coffee and tea intake with mortality: Prospective cohort study of UK Biobank participants *British Journal of Nutrition,* 129(1), 115-25

238   McDonald J, "Nutrition", A Symposium on Wine, Health and Society Institute, Washington. D.C. 24 February 1986

239   Paganga G, Miller N & Rice-Evans CA (1999) The polyphenolic content of fruit and vegetables and their antioxidant activities. What does a serving constitute?. *Free radical research*, *30*(2), 153-162.

240   Meng X et al (2020) "Health Benefits and Molecular Mechanisms of Resveratrol: A Narrative Review" *Foods* 9, no. 3: 340.

241   Ren B et al (2021) Resveratrol for cancer therapy: Challenges and future perspectives. *Cancer letters*, 515, 63-72.

242   Bhatt JK, Thomas S & Nanjan MJ (2012) Resveratrol supplementation improves glycemic control in type 2 diabetes mellitus. *Nutrition research*, 32(7), 537-541

243   Turner RS et al (2015) A randomized, double-blind, placebo-controlled trial of resveratrol for Alzheimer disease. *Neurology*, 85(16), 1383-1391.

244   Martínez L et al (2018) Hydroxytyrosol: Health Benefits and Use as Functional Ingredient in Meat. *Medicines (Basel)*. 23;5(1):13

245   Silva AFR et al (2020) Application of Hydroxytyrosol in the Functional Foods Field: From Ingredient to Dietary Supplements. *Antioxidants (Basel)* 8;9(12):1246

246   Gallardo-Fernández M et al (2022) Hydroxytyrosol in foods: Analysis, food sources, eu dietary intake, and potential uses. *Foods*, 11(15), 2355

247   Tuck KL et al (2001) The in vivo fate of hydroxytyrosol and tyrosol, antioxidant phenolic constituents of olive oil, after intravenous and oral dosing of labeled compounds to rats. *The Journal of nutrition*, 131(7), 1993-1996

248   Pérez-Mañá C et al (2015) Ethanol induces hydroxytyrosol formation in humans. *Pharmacological research*, 95, 27-33.

249   Arranz S et al (2012) Wine, beer, alcohol and polyphenols on cardiovascular disease and cancer. *Nutrients*, 4(7), 759-781.

250   Weissman G. (2010) *FASEB Journal*, 11 June

251   Cordova AC & Sumpio BE (2009) Polyphenols are medicine: Is it time to prescribe red wine for our patients? *The International journal of angiology*, 18(3), 111.

252   González PA et al (2022) Differences in the levels of sulphites and pesticide residues in soils and wines and under organic

and conventional production methods. *Journal of Food Composition and Analysis*, 112, 104714.

253   Silva M et al (2019) Sulfite concentration and the occurrence of headache in young adults: a prospective study. *Eur J Clin Nutr* 73, 1316–1322

254   Panconesi A (2008) Alcohol and migraine: trigger factor, consumption, mechanisms. A review *The journal of headache and pain* 9.1 : 19-27.

255   Vicini J L et al (2021). Residues of glyphosate in food and dietary exposure. *Comprehensive Reviews in Food Science and Food Safety*, *20*(5), 5226-5257.

256   Delmas MA et al (2016) Does organic wine taste better? An analysis of experts' ratings *Journal of Wine Economics* 11.3 : 329-354.

257   Soleas GJ & Goldberg DM (2000). Pesticide residues in unfermented grape juices and raw wines: a 5-year survey of more than 3000 products. *Journal of wine research*, 11(3), 197-207.

258   González PA et al (2022) Differences in the levels of sulphites and pesticide residues in soils and wines and under organic and conventional production methods. *Journal of Food Composition and Analysis*, 112, 104714

259   Reeve JR et al (2005) Soil and winegrape quality in biodynamically and organically managed vineyards *American journal of enology and viticulture* 56.4 : 367-376.

260   Döring J et al (2015). Ökologischer und biodynamischer Weinbau in der Forschung–Langzeitversuch INBIODYN.

261   Santoni M et al (2022) A review of scientific research on biodynamic agriculture. *Organic Agriculture* 12.3 : 373-396

262   Tassoni A et al (2013) Comparison of biogenic amine and polyphenol profiles of grape berries and wines obtained following conventional, organic and biodynamic agricultural and oenological practices. *Food Chemistry* 139.1-4 : 405-413.

263   Parpinello GP et al (2015) Chemical and sensory characterisation of Sangiovese red wines: Comparison between biodynamic and organic management. *Food Chemistry*, 167, 145-152.

264   Preti R et al (2016) Biogenic amine profiles and antioxidant properties of Italian red wines from different price categories. *Journal of Food Composition and Analysis*, 46, 7-14.

265   Sanlier N, Bektesoglu M (2021) Migraine and Biogenic Amines. *Annals of Medical and Health Sciences Research*, *11*(4).

266   Thun M (2010) "When Wine Tastes Best: A Biodynamic Calendar for Wine Drinkers" Floris Books

267   Parr WV et al (2017) Expectation or sensorial reality? An empirical investigation of the biodynamic calendar for wine drinkers. *PloS one*, 12(1), e0169257.

268   Parris M *The Spectator,* 21 Jan 2017

269   Orwell G (1933) "Down and out in Paris and London"

270   WCRF-AICR Food, Nutrition, Physical Activity and the Prevention of Cancer 2007

271   Kiviniemia TO et al (2007) Atherosclerosis Volume 195, Issue 2, e176-e181

272   Kiviniemi TO et al (2009) High dose of red wine elicits enhanced inhibition of bhasfibrinolysis. *European Journal of Preventive Cardiology* 16.2 : 161-163.

273   Naissides M et al (2006) The effect of chronic consumption of red wine on cardiovascular disease risk factors in postmenopausal women. *Atherosclerosis*, 185(2), 438-445

274   McAnulty LS et al (2019). Chronic and acute effects of red wine versus red muscadine grape juice on body composition, blood lipids, vascular performance, inflammation, and antioxidant capacity in overweight adults. *International Journal of Wine Research*, 13-22.

275   Imhof A et al (2009) Effect of drinking on adiponectin in healthy men and women: a randomized intervention study of water, ethanol, red wine, and beer with or without alcohol. *Diabetes Care*, 32(6), 1101-1103.

276   Chiva-Blanch G et al (2013) Effects of Wine, Alcohol and Polyphenols on Cardiovascular Disease Risk Factors: Evidence from Human Studies *Alcohol and Alcoholism* 48 (3), 270-277

277   Chiva-Blanch G et al (2013) Effects of red wine polyphenols and alcohol on glucose metabolism and the lipid profile: A randomized clinical trial *Clinical Nutrition*, 32(2), 200 - 206

278   Kronenberg F et al. (2022) Lipoprotein(a) in atherosclerotic cardiovascular disease and aortic stenosis: a European Atherosclerosis Society consensus statement. *Eur Heart J.* 43(39):3925-3946.

279   Lian C (1915) L'alcoholisme, cause d'hypertension arterielle *Bull Acad Natl Med (Paris)*

280   Chiva-Blanch G et al. Dealcoholized red wine decreases systolic and diastolic blood pressure and increases plasma nitric oxide. *Circulation research* 111.8 (2012): 1065-1068.

281   Queipo-Ortuño MI et al (2012). Influence of red wine polyphenols and ethanol on the gut microbiota ecology and biochemical biomarkers. *The American journal of clinical nutrition*, 95(6), 1323-1334.

282   De la Torre R et al (2006) Is dopamine behind the health benefits of red wine? *Eur J Nutr* 45:307–310

283   Pérez-Mañá C et al (2015) Moderate consumption of wine, through both its phenolic compounds and alcohol content, promotes hydroxytyrosol endogenous generation in humans. A randomized controlled trial. *Molecular nutrition & food research* 59.6 : 1213-1216

284   De La Torre R et al (2006) op.cit.

285   Mezue K et al (2023) Reduced stress-related neural network activity mediates the effect of alcohol on cardiovascular risk. *Journal of the American College of Cardiology*, 81(24), 2315-2325.

286   pers.comm. August 2022

287   Stasi A et al (2014). Italian consumers' preferences regarding dealcoholized wine, information and price. *Wine Economics and Policy*, 3(1), 54-61.

288   *Science Daily* 14 July 2021

289   *Daily Telegraph* 27 July 2021

290   Kroeger CM et al (2018) Scientific rigor and credibility in the nutrition research landscape. *The American journal of clinical nutrition*, 107(3), 484-494.

291   Shankar P, Ahuja S & Sriram K. (2013). Non-nutritive sweeteners: review and update. *Nutrition*, 29(11-12), 1293-1299.

292   Kearns CE et al (2016) Sugar industry and coronary heart disease research: a historical analysis of internal industry documents. *JAMA internal medicine*, 176(11), 1680-1685.

293   Vos M et al (2020) Exploring the influence of alcohol industry funding in observational studies on moderate alcohol consumption and health. *Advances in Nutrition*, 11(5), 1384-1391.

294   *New York Times* 18 June 2018.

295   Dawber TR (2013) The Framingham Study. *Harvard University Press*

296   Wood AM et al (2018) Risk thresholds for alcohol consumption: combined analysis of individual-participant data for 599,912 current drinkers in 83 prospective studies. *The Lancet* 391.10129 (1513-1523).

297   Stockwell T et al (2016) Do "Moderate" Drinkers Have Reduced Mortality Risk? A Systematic Review and Meta-Analysis of Alcohol Consumption and All-Cause Mortality *Journal of Studies on Alcohol and Drugs,* 77(2), 185-198

298   Topiwala A et al (2022) Alcohol consumption and telomere length: Mendelian randomization clarifies alcohol's effects. *Molecular Psychiatry*, 27(10), 4001-4008

299   *The Times* 26 July 2022

300   Gomes NM et al (2011) Comparative biology of mammalian telomeres: hypotheses on ancestral states and the roles of telomeres in longevity determination. *Aging Cell.* 10 (5): 761–8

301   Dixit S et al (2019) Alcohol consumption and leukocyte telomere length. *Scientific reports*, 9(1), 1404.

302   Gambini J et al (2021) Moderate red wine consumption increases the expression of longevity-associated genes in controlled human populations and extends lifespan in Drosophila melanogaster. *Antioxidants*, 10(2), 301

303   Freitas-Simoes TM, Ros E & Sala-Vila A (2016) Nutrients, foods, dietary patterns and telomere length: Update of epidemiological studies and randomized trials. *Metabolism*, 65(4), 406-415.

304   Hydes TJ et al (2019) A comparison of gender-linked population cancer risks between alcohol and tobacco: how many cigarettes are there in a bottle of wine? *BMC Public Health* 19, 316

305   Millwood IY et al (2019) Conventional and genetic evidence on alcohol and vascular disease aetiology: a prospective study of 500,000 men and women in China. *The Lancet*, 393(10183), 1831-1842

306   "Canada's Guidance on Alcohol and Health: Final Report" January 2023

307   Goebbels J.   Address to "Hochschule für Politik", 9th January 1928

308   McGuire S (2016) Scientific Report of the 2015 Dietary Guidelines Advisory Committee Washington, DC: US Departments of Agriculture and Health and Human Services, 2015. *Adv Nutr.* 15;7(1):202-4.

309   Davies S reported in *Daily Mail* 8 January 2016

310   "UK Chief Medical Officers' Low Risk Drinking Guidelines" August 2016

311   Snowdon C *Sunday Times* 29 Oct 2017.

312   Jin M et al (2013) Alcohol drinking and all cancer mortality: a meta-analysis. *Annals of oncology* 24.3 : 807-816

313   Seitz H K & Becker P (2007) Alcohol metabolism and cancer risk. *Alcohol Research & Health*, 30(1), 38.

314   Halsted CH et al (2002) Metabolic interactions of alcohol and folate. *The Journal of nutrition*, 132(8), 2367S-2372S.

315   Scaglione F & Panzavolta G (2014) Folate, folic acid and 5-methyltetrahydrofolate are not the same thing. *Xenobiotica*, 44(5), 480-488.

316   Baglietto L et al (2005). Does dietary folate intake modify effect of alcohol consumption on breast cancer risk? Prospective cohort study. *BMJ*, 331(7520), 807.

317   Ozaras R et al (2003). N-acetylcysteine attenuates alcohol-induced oxidative stress in the rat. *World journal of gastroenterology*, 9(1), 125.

318   Morley KC et al (2018). N-acetyl cysteine in the treatment of alcohol use disorder in patients with liver disease: Rationale for further research. *Expert opinion on investigational drugs*, 27(8), 667-675.

319   Martinotti G et al (2010) Acetyl-L-carnitine for alcohol craving and relapse prevention in anhedonic alcoholics: a randomized, double-blind, placebo-controlled pilot trial. *Alcohol & Alcoholism,* 45(5), 449-455.

320   Giovinazzo G et al (2019) Wine Polyphenols and Health. *Refer. Ser. Phytochem.* 1135–1155.

321   Boban M et al (2016) Drinking pattern of wine and effects on human health: *Food Funct.* 7, 2937-2942

322   Gea A et al (2014) Mediterranean alcohol-drinking pattern and mortality in the SUN Project: a prospective cohort study. *Br J Nutr.*111(10):1871-80.

323   Rukmini AV et al (2021) Circadian regulation of breath alcohol concentration. *Sleep*, 44(6), zsaa270.

324   Hisler GC et al (2021) Is there a 24-hour rhythm in alcohol craving and does it vary by sleep/circadian timing? *Chronobiol Int.*;38(1):109-121

325   Jensen MK et al (2002) Alcoholic beverage preference and risk of becoming a heavy drinker. *Epidemiology*, 127-132.

326   Smart R G & Walsh G (1999). Heavy drinking and problems among wine drinkers. *Journal of studies on alcohol*, 60(4), 467-471.

327   Esser MB et al (2014) Prevalence of alcohol dependence among US adult drinkers, 2009–2011. *Preventing chronic disease*, 11.

328   Dube SR et al (2002) Adverse childhood experiences and personal alcohol abuse as an adult. *Addictive behaviors*, 27(5), 713-725

329 Šulejová K et al (2022). Relationship between alcohol consumption and adverse childhood experiences in college students – A cross-sectional study. *Frontiers in psychology*, 13, 1004651.

330   Guilford JM & Pezzuto JM (2011) Wine and health: A review. *American Journal of Enology and Viticulture*, 62(4), 471-486.

331   Snopek L et al (2018) Contribution of red wine consumption to human health protection *Molecules*, 23(7), 1684.

332   Maskarinec G (2009) Cancer protective properties of cocoa: a review of the epidemiologic evidence. *Nutrition and Cancer*, 61(5), 573-579

333   Lim RR et al (2022) Gut microbiome responses to dietary intervention with hypocholesterolemic vegetable oils. *npj Biofilms and Microbiomes*, 8(1)

334   WHO website, August 2023

335   Hillman RS & Steinberg SE (1982) The effects of alcohol on folate metabolism. *Annual review of medicine*, 33(1), 345-354

336   Sharma J & Krupenko SA (2020). Folate pathways mediating the effects of ethanol in tumorigenesis. *Chemico-biological interactions*, 324, 109091

337   Ferenczi EA et al (2010) Can a statin neutralize the cardiovascular risk of unhealthy dietary choices?. *The American Journal of Cardiology,* 106(4), 587-592.

338   (2023) Effectiveness of non-pharmaceutical interventions to reduce transmission of COVID-19 in the UK, *UK Health Security Agency*

339   Smith R (2011) Battling over safe alcohol limits, *BMJ blogs* 14 Nov

340   Teicholz N (2015) The scientific report guiding the US dietary guidelines: is it scientific?. *BMJ*, 351, h4962.

INDEX

37224764R00101